Contents

Preface   v

Part 1. All the Stuff You Never Wanted to Think About   1

Questions 1–10 describe the anatomy of the penis, define erectile dysfunction, and discuss some of the causes of erectile dysfunction.
- What is erectile dysfunction?
- What causes erectile dysfunction?
- Is erectile dysfunction or sexual dysfunction a normal process of aging?
- Is erectile dysfunction curable?

Part 2. Evaluating Erectile Dysfunction: What to Expect   33

Questions 11–25 describe the kinds of questions and tests that your doctor may use to determine what might be causing erectile dysfunction.
- What questions might the doctor ask me during my initial visit?
- What is the doctor looking for during the physical examination?
- What happens after the history, physical examination, and laboratory tests have been carried out?
- What laboratory tests are performed?

Part 3. What Are the Other Types of Sexual Dysfunction?   53

Questions 26–32 discuss other forms of sexual dysfunction that can be related to erectile dysfunction.
- What is retrograde ejaculation and what causes it?
- What is priapism and prolonged erection?
- What is Peyronie's disease and what causes it?

Part 4. Treatment   61

Questions 33–85 discuss various options for treating erectile dysfunction, along with possible side effects and complications.
- What are the current treatment options for erectile dysfunction?

- What are the benefits and risks of testosterone therapy?
- How does Viagra compare to other therapies?
- What is the success rate of MUSE?
- What is a penile prosthesis?
- What is penile bypass surgery and who is a candidate?
- What are the investigational therapies and how can I try one of these?
- Can I combine therapies?

Part 5. Talking About and Living With Erectile Dysfunction   155

Questions 86–100 address the relationship and lifestyle issues that erectile dysfunction and its treatment can cause. Question 100 offers resources for more information.

- I am embarrassed about my erectile troubles and have found myself avoiding my wife/partner. How do I discuss this with my partner/wife?
- If I don't have a primary care provider, who should I see to have my erectile dysfunction evaluated and treated?
- Is there a role for sex therapy in the treatment of erectile dysfunction?
- Does insurance cover a penile prosthesis?
- I have angina. Is sex bad for me?

Glossary   177

Appendix A   189

Appendix B   193

Index   195

Why, you might ask, would someone—or in this case, two individuals—want to write a book on erectile dysfunction? Haven't the media thoroughly covered this topic? Despite the extensive media coverage of sildenafil (Viagra), the oral therapy for erectile dysfunction, the discussion of erectile dysfunction by prominent figures, and the feeling that there is a growing level of comfort with discussing erectile dysfunction, this issue still remains a source of anxiety and frustration for both patients and physicians. This is probably best reflected by the fact that before the advent of "the little blue pill," only 10% of men with erectile dysfunction sought help for this problem. Even though oral therapy is now readily available, however, only 20% seek evaluation and treatment for their erectile dysfunction.

There are probably many reasons, both physician- and patient-related, for the low numbers of men seeking treatment. Not all men with erectile dysfunction are willing to bring up this subject with their doctors. Similarly, not all physicians feel comfortable talking about erectile function and sexuality, nor are they comfortable treating erectile dysfunction. Cultural, religious, societal, and personal issues may prevent open discussion, but it is also a problem of education: Many people simply don't realize how widespread this problem is and, therefore, think of it as "abnormal."

We should not forget that erectile dysfunction is primarily a *couple's* problem. In other words, with each case of erectile dysfunction, both the patient *and his partner* are unable to share sexual intercourse. Thus, when we say that "50% of men older than the age of 40 years have some degree of erectile dysfunction," we really mean that "50% of couples that include a man older than the age of 40 years are affected." The potential magnitude of this problem, its effects on both individuals in the relationship, and the difficulty in discussing erectile dysfunction are what prompted us to take on this task.

This book was written by a urologist who treats men with erectile dysfunction, and contributed to by a patient who has personal experience with many of the treatments for erectile dysfunction.

The Doctor

My name is Pamela Ellsworth, and I am a urologist. I did a pediatric urology fellowship after completing my urology residency but stumbled into the field of erectile dysfunction when I chose to return to Dartmouth–Hitchcock Medical Center in Hanover, New Hampshire. I had a big assignment: I was to replace a well-respected and cherished mentor, Dr. John Richardson, who ran the erectile dysfunction clinic. Luckily, I had trained with Dr. Richardson and had the basics down pat. As anyone would do when faced with the "unknown," I quickly purchased several texts, signed up for instructional courses, and kept my eyes and ears open for any information on erectile dysfunction that was available. I had some tough shoes to fill, as Dr. Richardson was highly regarded by virtually all of his patients—who now had a *female* urologist taking over his work.

Some of you may be wondering why a woman would want to go into a male-dominated and -oriented discipline. Of course, one could wonder the same about why men enter the field of obstetrics and gynecology. Ultimately, something just draws you to the subject. I have never regretted my decision to enter this field. Have I filled Dr. Richardson's shoes? I don't know—that's a question that my patients must answer. However, I have found the treatment of erectile dysfunction to be the most rewarding aspect of my adult urology practice. How often, I ask myself, can other specialists improve the quality of life for two individuals—both the patient and his partner?

The Patient

My name is Bob Stanley, and I am the "patient." I experienced what the medical community calls "erectile dysfunction." No, it doesn't mean that I am some sort of lurking deviant, or a person who experiments with the sexual occult. Simply stated, in my case, it meant that I could no longer participate completely in sexual intercourse.

I am an average man, married more than 30 years to Victoria, with what I think was a normal husband-and-wife relationship. We enjoyed sex, although in recent years the frequency had decreased to once or twice per month. Was this average? Who knows? I'm not Dr. Kinsey! But it seemed to satisfy us. We had two grown children who were now on their own, and we were settling into the phase of life called "early retirement." During my career, I had been an insurance executive at one of the large corporations in Hartford, Connecticut. Victoria and I moved to Vermont after retiring, living in an area locally called the "upper valley," an idyllic greensward along the Connecticut River, straddling New Hampshire and Vermont. One of the largest employers in the area is Dartmouth–Hitchcock Medical Center, a teaching hospital that is affiliated with Dartmouth Medical School.

This proximity to the medical center seemed to work out well for us, because I had been diagnosed with diabetes mellitus and Victoria had been treated for breast cancer. We felt that it would be nice to be near a first-class medical facility, given these circumstances. Still, in our naïveté, we thought we would hardly need this center, using it only for the occasional checkup or flu shot. Unfortunately, we had not taken into consideration how the future would affect us. In any event, it was shortly after we moved north that I experienced a decrease in my sexual function. Over a 1-year stretch, I noticed that I had difficulty achieving and maintaining an erection. Was it the diabetes? Was it my age? (I was now well into my sixties.) Or was it merely psychological? I didn't know at the time.

Over an 8-year period, I tried a number of therapeutic remedies for my erectile dysfunction, including injection therapy, the vacuum device, and eventually the placement of a penile prosthesis into my body. In this book, I will periodically comment on these treatments from my perspective as a patient. This road has not been an easy one, and I will try to share with you (if you will excuse the expression) the "ups and downs," the frustrations and indignities that I encountered, and—oh yes—my successes. It is my intention to provide the "humanistic" aspect of the evaluation and management of erectile dysfunction, while Dr. Ellsworth addresses the more concrete medical issues—the causes, evaluation, and management of erectile dysfunction.

100 Questions & Answers About Erectile Dysfunction

Second Edition

Pamela Ellsworth, MD

Associate Professor of Surgery
Department of Urology
Brown University Medical Center
Providence, RI

JONES AND BARTLETT PUBLISHERS

Sudbury, Massachusetts

BOSTON   TORONTO   LONDON   SINGAPORE

World Headquarters

Jones and Bartlett Publishers	Jones and Bartlett Publishers	Jones and Bartlett Publishers
40 Tall Pine Drive	Canada	International
Sudbury, MA 01776	6339 Ormindale Way	Barb House, Barb Mews
978-443-5000	Mississauga, Ontario	London W6 7PA
info@jbpub.com	L5V 1J2	UK
www.jbpub.com	CANADA	

Jones and Bartlett's books and products are available through most bookstores and online booksellers. To contact Jones and Bartlett Publishers directly, call 800-832-0034, fax 978-443-8000, or visit our website www.jbpub.com.

Substantial discounts on bulk quantities of Jones and Bartlett's publications are available to corporations, professional associations,and other qualified organizations. For details and specific discount information, contact the special sales department at Jones and Bartlett via the above contact information or send an email to specialsales@jbpub.com.

Copyright © 2008 by Jones and Bartlett Publishers, Inc.
ISBN 13: 978-0-7637-53573
ISBN 10: 0-7637-53572
Cover images: Couple © digitalskillet/Shutterstock, Inc.; Young man © MaxFX/Shutterstock, Inc.; Mature man © Steve Luker/Shutterstock, Inc.

The authors, editor, and publisher have made every effort to provide accurate information. However, they are not responsible for errors, omissions, or for any outcomes related to the use of the contents of this book and take no responsibility for the use of the products and procedures described. Treatments and side effects described in this book may not be applicable to all people; likewise, some people may require a dose or experience a side effect that is not described herein. Drugs and medical devices are discussed that may have limited availability controlled by the Food and Drug Administration (FDA) for use only in a research study or clinical trial. Research, clinical practice, and government regulations often change the accepted standard in this field. When consideration is being given to use of any drug in the clinical setting, the health care provider or reader is responsible for determining FDA status of the drug, reading the package insert, and reviewing prescribing information for the most up-to-date recommendations on dose, precautions, and contraindications, and determining the appropriate usage for the product. This is especially important in the case of drugs that are new or seldom used.

CIP Data for this text was not available at the time of printing

6048

Production Credits
Executive Editor: Christopher Davis
Production Director: Amy Rose
Associate Production Editor: Rachel Rossi
Associate Editor: Kathy Richardson
Associate Marketing Manager: Rebecca Wasley
Manufacturing Buyer: Therese Connell
Composition: Appingo
Cover Design: Jon Ayotte
Printing and Binding: Malloy, Inc.
Cover Printing: Malloy, Inc.

Printed in the United States of America
11 10 09 08 07   10 9 8 7 6 5 4 3 2 1

All the Stuff You Never Wanted to Think About

1. How do erections normally occur?

More ...

1. How do erections normally occur?

Erection

The process whereby the penis becomes rigid.

Penis

The male organ that is used for urination and intercourse.

Corpora cavernosa

Two cylindrical structures in the penis that are composed of the penile erectile tissue. They are located on the top of the penis. (singular: corpus cavernosum)

Corpus spongiosum

One of the three cylindrical structures in the penis. The urethra passes through the corpus spongiosum. It is not involved in erections.

Glans

The tip of the penis.

Tunica albuginea

Dense, fibrous, elastic sheath enclosing the corpora cavernosa in the penis. Compression of small veins against the tunica albuginea during erection holds back outflow of blood from the corpora, causing the penis to be rigid.

In order to understand how an **erection** (rigidity of the penis) occurs, one must first learn a little about the anatomy of the **penis**. The penis may look like one simple tube, but it is actually composed of three cylinders. There are two on the top of the penis called the **corpora cavernosa** (a Latin phrase meaning, roughly, "bodies composed of hollows or caves") and one on the underside of the penis, the **corpus spongiosum** ("sponge-like body") (Figure 1). The tip of the penis, called the **glans,** is part of the corpus spongiosum. The corpora cavernosa are surrounded by a fibroelastic layer of tissue, the **tunica albuginea** (literally, "white coat," referring to the fact that the tunica albuginea is a thick white membrane wrapped around the corpora cavernosa like a cloak). The two corpora cavernosa contain numerous compartments that are filled with blood during sexual excitement, which is what makes the penis become erect. The corpus spongiosum contains the **urethra,** the tube that one urinates through, and it is not involved in the erectile process.

The two corpora cavernosa and the corpus spongiosum each have an **artery** (a blood vessel that carries oxygenated blood from the heart to other parts of the body) that supplies it. The artery to each corpus cavernosum runs through its center (Figure 2). The two corpora cavernosa communicate in the middle of the penis, thus allowing blood from one corpus cavernosum to flow into the other. The veins that drain the penis are also different for the corpus spongiosum and the corpora cavernosa. (A **vein** is a blood vessel that carries deoxygenated blood from the tissues back to the heart.) The veins that drain the corpora cavernosa, unlike the

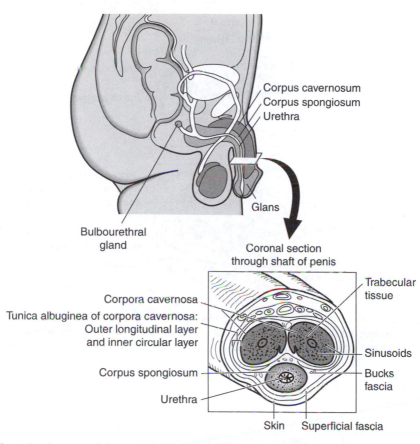

Corpus cavernosum
Corpus spongiosum
Urethra

Glans

Bulbourethral
gland

Coronal section
through shaft of penis

Trabecular
tissue

Corpora cavernosa

Tunica albuginea of corpora cavernosa:
Outer longitudinal layer
and inner circular layer

Sinusoids

Corpus spongiosum

Bucks
fascia

Urethra

Skin   Superficial fascia

Figure 1   Anatomy of the penis. Reprinted with permission from Br J Urol Intl 2001; 88(Suppl 3):3–10.

arteries, run along the outer edge of the corpora caver-nosa, just underneath the tunica albuginea (Figure 2).

So why are all these veins and arteries important? Here's why: when a man becomes aroused, his brain and the nerves in his pelvis release chemicals that increase blood flow into the penis. The corpora cavernosa are similar to a sponge: just as a sponge absorbs liquids into its air spaces and distends when submerged, the

Urethra

The tube that one urinates through.

Artery

A blood vessel that carries oxygenated blood from the heart to other parts of the body.

Vein

A blood vessel in the body that carries deoxygenated blood from the tissues back to the heart.

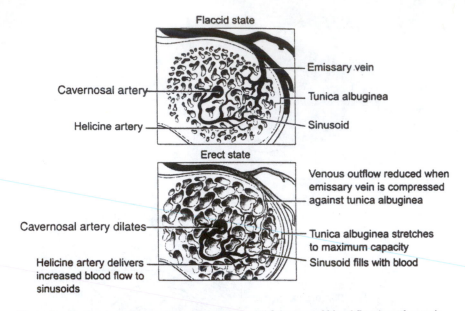

Figure 2 Mechanism of normal erectile response. With increased blood flow into the penis, there is compression of the veins, leading to decreased outflow. The penis becomes filled with blood and expands into an erection. Reprinted with permission from Br J Urol Intl 2001; 88(Suppl 3):3–10.

Sinusoid

A blood-filled cavernous space. In the penis, these spaces are separated by a network of connective tissues containing muscle cells, small arteries, veins, and nerves.

Nerve

A cordlike structure composed of a collection of nerve fibers that conveys impulses between a part of the central nervous system and some other region of the body.

corpora cavernosa have hollow spaces, or **sinusoids**, that distend with blood when sexual excitement causes increased blood flow to the penis. As the sinusoids fill with blood and distend, they compress the veins against the tunica albuginea. It is this compression of the veins that prevents blood from draining out of the penis, which promotes full rigidity and maintenance of the rigidity (Figure 2).

You might be surprised to learn that erections are not simply something that happens in the penis. For an erection to occur, there must be proper functioning of many physical structures and systems: the brain, certain **nerves** (cordlike structures that convey impulses between the central nervous system and some other part of the body) in the **pelvis** (the part of the body that is framed by the hip bones), and the arteries and veins that supply the penis. When a man is aroused, the brain tells special nerves in the pelvis to release chemicals called **neurotransmitters**, which in turn stimulate the blood vessels in the penis to open up and the smooth muscle in the corpora cavernosa to relax to increase blood flow into the penis. After sexual performance is completed, the brain releases other chemicals that tell the arteries in the penis to constrict, thus decreasing blood flow to the penis and allowing the veins to drain the blood out of the penis (see Question 4 and Figure 4 for more details). These chemicals that cause constriction of smooth muscle may also be released during times of stress and may adversely affect erectile function.

Now that you know that the erectile process is a neurovascular event, then it becomes clear that any disease process that affects the brain, the nerves in the pelvis, the arteries to and within the penis, the veins in the penis, the tunica albuginea, or the "erectile tissue" within the corpora cavernosa may affect erectile function.

2. What is erectile dysfunction?

The National Institutes of Health (NIH) definition of **erectile dysfunction**, previously called **impotence**, is *the consistent inability to achieve and/or maintain an erection*

Pelvis

The part of the body that is framed by the hip bones.

Neurotransmitter

A chemical released from a nerve cell that transmits an impulse to another nerve, cell, or organ.

For an erection to occur, there must be proper functioning of many physical structures and systems.

Erectile dysfunction

The inability to achieve and/or maintain an erection satisfactory for the completion of sexual performance.

Impotence

See *erectile dysfunction.*

Many men may experience temporary erection problems at some point in their lives due to stress, alcohol use, or psychological problems.

Subjective

Pertaining to or perceived by the affected individual, but not perceptible to the other senses of another person.

Objective

Perceptible to the external senses; something the physician uses to quantify, measure, or identify.

Nocturnal

Occurring or active at night.

Sexual dysfunction

An abnormality in function of any component of the sexual response cycle, libido, arousal (erection), climax/ejaculation, detumescence.

satisfactory for the completion of sexual performance. Many men may experience temporary erection problems at some point in their lives due to stress, alcohol use, or psychological problems, but such occasional problems do not mean that erectile dysfunction will become a chronic condition. It is also important to remember that the mind has very powerful effects, and a man can sabotage his erections just by worrying about his ability to perform, even when no physical problem exists. That is why one of the key components of the definition of erectile dysfunction is that it is a *persistent* or *continuous* problem. Looking carefully at this definition, you can see that it is a **subjective** definition, meaning that the individual (and/or his partner) is the person who decides that his erections are not satisfactory. This is in comparison to an **objective** definition, in which an observer or a test makes the decision that the erection is not satisfactory. The definition is not an all-or-nothing one, meaning that different men may experience different degrees of erectile dysfunction. The most severe form of erectile dysfunction would be the complete absence of erections—no **nocturnal** (nighttime) erections, morning erections, or erections noted with stimulation; milder forms may be associated with inadequate degree or duration of rigidity.

Erectile dysfunction is a form of sexual dysfunction. The term **sexual dysfunction** applies to a variety of problems with sex, so the two terms are not really interchangeable (see Question 8). It is important that you determine early in your visit with your doctor whether your problem is erectile dysfunction and not another type of sexual dysfunction.

Erectile dysfunction is not a **disease** in and of itself; rather, it is a manifestation of an underlying medical condition. It is important to evaluate men with erectile dysfunction to identify the underlying disease process(es) that is causing this problem because it may be a **symptom** (i.e., subjective evidence) of a condition that could cause the individual further harm. In addition, by treating the underlying disease processes, one may hopefully prevent further progression of the erectile dysfunction.

Disease

Any change from or interruption of the normal structure or function of any part or organ.

Symptom

Subjective evidence of a disease, i.e., something the patient describes, such as pain in abdomen.

3. How common is erectile dysfunction?

The Massachusetts Male Aging Study was probably the first study that brought to light how common erectile dysfunction is. This study demonstrated that 52% of men between the ages of 40 and 70 have some degree of erectile dysfunction (Figure 3). Of those individuals, 10% noted complete erectile dysfunction,

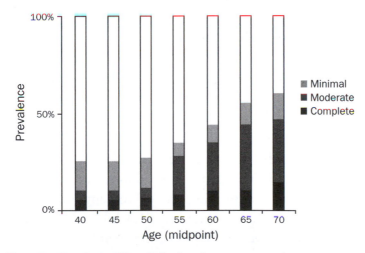

Figure 3   Prevalence of Erectile Dysfunction.
Source: Adapted with permission from Feldman, HA, Goldstein I, Hatzichristou DG, Krane RJ and McKinlay JB: Impotence and its medical and psychological correlates: results of the Massachusetts Male Aging Study. *J Urol* 1994; 151: 54–61.

25% noted moderate erectile dysfunction, and most noted mild erectile dysfunction.

In the United States, approximately 50 million men suffer from erectile dysfunction. The **prevalence** (number of cases of a disease that are present at a given point in time) of erectile dysfunction is age dependent, with the rate of complete erectile dysfunction increasing from 5% among men 40 years old to 15% among those 70 years old. As our population continues to grow and age, we can only expect this number to increase. The worldwide prevalence of erectile dysfunction was 152 million in 1995 and is expected to increase to 322 million in 2025. Much of this increase will occur in the developing world and reflects the aging of the world's population.

The **incidence** (i.e., the number of new cases occurring during a specific period of time) of erectile dysfunction is higher in men with certain diseases, such as diabetes mellitus, hypertension, cardiovascular disease, spinal cord injury, and **hypercholesterolemia** (high cholesterol levels) (see Question 4).

The potential economic impact of erectile dysfunction is huge. In the 1985 National Ambulatory Medical Care Survey, erectile dysfunction was associated with 525,000 outpatient office visits, and the 1995 National Hospital Discharge Survey reported that it accounted for more than 30,000 hospital admissions. The projected sales of Viagra, the first oral therapy for erectile dysfunction, were estimated at $1.4 billion for 1999. Who should cover the costs of the treatment of erectile dysfunction remains a source of debate.

Prevalence

The number of cases of a disease that are present in a population at one given point in time.

Incidence

The rate at which a certain event occurs, e.g., the number of new cases of a specific disease occurring during a certain period.

Hypercholester-olemia

Elevated cholesterol levels.

4. What causes erectile dysfunction?

Many medical conditions and medications (Table 1) can cause erectile dysfunction. Smoking, alcohol abuse, drug abuse, stress, and **depression** can also cause erectile dysfunction. Considering erectile function as a neurovascular event, we can divide the causes of erectile dysfunction into those that affect the brain and nerves (**neurologic**) and those that affect the arteries and veins (**vascular**).

Depression

A mental state of depressed mood characterized by feelings of sadness, despair, and discouragement.

Neurologic Conditions That Cause Erectile Dysfunction

A variety of neurologic conditions can cause erectile dysfunction. The most common of these are spinal cord injury, lumbar disk disease, stroke, Parkinson's disease, multiple sclerosis, Alzheimer's disease, and pituitary disease (pituitary **adenoma**). In addition, certain surgical procedures, such as radical prostatectomy for prostate cancer and surgery for rectal cancer, can injure the pelvic nerves. The incidence of erectile dysfunction after radical prostatectomy varies according to whether the patient experienced erectile dysfunction before surgery and whether a nerve-sparing procedure was performed. Reported rates of erectile dysfunction after bilateral nerve-sparing radical prostatectomy range from 18% to 82%. Other factors unrelated to disease or surgery can also cause erectile dysfunction. For example, long-distance bicycle riding on bicycles with small, hard seats has been implicated as a cause of erectile dysfunction, possibly by nerve or vascular compression.

Neurologic

Pertaining to the brain and nerves.

Vascular

Pertaining to blood vessels.

Adenoma

A benign, noncancerous tumor in which the cells form glandular structures.

Table 1 Medications Associated with Erectile Dysfunction

acebutolol
acetazolarnide
alimemazine
allopurinol
aiprazolarn
aiprenolol
alseroxylon
alufibrate
amiloride
amoxapine
amphetamine
anisotropine
arniodarone
arnitriptytine
atenolol
atropine
aurothioglucose
azathioprine
baclofen
bendrofluazide
   (bendroflumethi-
   azide)
benperidol
benzatropine
benzbromarone
benzhexol
benzphetamine
benztropine
betamethasone
betaxolol
bethanidine
bezafibrate
biperiden
bisoprolol
bopindolol
bornaprine
bromocriptine
bromperidol
broniazepam
brotizolam
bumetanide
bunitrolol
bupranolol
buprenorphine

buserelin
buspirone
busuiphan (busul-
   fan)
butaperazine
butizide
butobarbitone
   (butobarbital)
camazepam
camylofin
canrenoate-K
captopril
carazolol
carbamazepine
carteolol
celiprolol
chlordiazepoxide
chloroquine
chlorphentermine
chlorpromazine
chlorprothixene
chlorthalidone
choline theofyllinate
cimetidine
cinnarizine
clobazam
clofibrate
clomipramine
clonazepam
clonidine
clopenthixol
clozepam
cortisol
cortisone acetate
cyclobarbitone
   (cyclobarbital)
cyclobenzaprine
cyclospotin A
cyproterone
dantrolene
deserpidine
desipramine
desmethylim-
   ipramine

dexamethasone
dexamphetamine
   (dextroampheta-
   mine)
dextromoramide
dextropropoxyphene
diazepam
dibenzepin
dichlorphenamide
diclofenac
dicyclomine
diethyipropion
digoxin
dihydralazine
dihydroergotamine
dimenhydrinate
diphenhydramine
disopyramide
disulfiram
dixyrazine
dosulepin
doxepin
doxylamine
droperidol
enalapril
ephedrine
ergotamine
ethionamide
etofibrate
famotidine
felodipine
fenflutamine
fenofibrate
finasteride
flecainide
fluanisone
flunarizine
flunitrazepam
fluocortolone
fluoxetine
flupenrixol
fluphenaine
flurazepam
fluspirilene

flutamide
fluvoxamine
gemfibrozil
gestagenen
gestonoron caproate
glutethimide
glycopyrrolate
glycopyrronium
   bromide
goserelin
guanabenz
guanadrel
guanethidine
guanfacine
guanidine
guanoclot
guanoxan
haloperidol
hexamethonium
homatropine
hydantoins
hydralazine
hydrochlorothiazide
hydrocortisone
   dimorphone
   (hydromorphone)
hydroxychloroquine
hydroxyproges-
   terone
hydroxyzine
hyoscyamine
imipramine
indapamide
indomethacin
interferon
iodide
iproniazid
isocarboxazid
isoniazid
isopropamide
itraconazole
ketamine

(continued)

Table 1 (continued)

ketanserin
ketazolam
ketoconazole
labetalol
leuprolide
levomepromazine
lisinopril
lithium
lofepramine
lorazepam
loxapine
maprotiline
mazindol
mebanazine
mecamylamine
medroxyproges-
    terone
melperon
mepenzolate
mepindolol
meprobamate
mesoridazine
mesterolone
rnetaclazepam
methadilazin
methadone
rnethamphetamine
methantheline
methaqualone
methazolamide
methotrexate
methyldopa
methylphenobarbi-
    tone (methylphe-
    nobarbital)
methylprednisolone
methyltestosterone
methysergide
metipranolol
metixene
metoclopramide
metoprolol
metronidazole
metyrosine
mexiletine
midazolam

minoxidil
moclobemide
morphine
nadolol
naltrexone
naproxen
nifedipine
nitrendipine
nittazepam
nizatidine
nordazepam
norerhandrolone
norethisterone
    (norethindrone)
norlutin
nortripryline
oestrogens
omeprazole
opipramol
orphenadrine
oxazepam
oxazolam
oxprenolol
oxybutinin
    (oxybutynin)
oxycodone
oxymetazoline
oxypertine
oxyphencyclimine
oxyphenonium
paramethasone
pargyline
paroxetine
penbutolol
pentazocine
pentobarbitone
    (pentobarbital)
perazine
perhexiline
pericyaine
perphenazine
pethidine
    (meperidine)
phencyclidine
phendimetrazine
phenelzine

phenmetrazine
    (phendime-
    trazine)
phenobarbitone
    (phenobarbital)
phenoxybenzamine
phenrermine
phenylephrine
phenytoin
phenyl-
    propanolamine
pimozide
pindolol
pipamperone
pipoxolan
pirenzepine
piritramide
pizorifen
poldine
polyrhiazide
pramiverine
prazepam
prazosin
prednisolone
prednisone
prednylidene
pridinol
primidone
probucol
prochlorperazine
procyclidine
progesterone
proguanil
prolonium
    iodide
promazine
promethazine
propafenone
propanolol
propantheline
prorriptyline
prothipendyl
protionamide
pseudoephedrine
quinalbarbirone
    (secobarbital)

ramipril
ranitidine
rauwolfia
reserpine hyoscine
    (scopolamine)
selegiline
simvastatin
soralol
spironolactone
stilboestrol
    (diethylstilbestrol)
sulpiride
tamoxifen
temazepam
terazosin
testosterone
thiabendazole
thiazinamium
thiethylperazine
thiorhixene
thioridazine
tilidine
timolol
tranylcypromine
trazodone
triamcinolone
triazolam
trichlorrnerhiazide
rridihexethyl
trifluoperazine
trifluperidol
triflupromazine
trihexyphenidyl
trimeprazine
trimetaphan
trimipramine
triptorelin
trospium chloride
verapamil
vincristine
vinylbitone
    (vinylbital)
zopiclone
zuclopenthixol

Vascular Conditions That Cause Erectile Dysfunction

From a vascular standpoint, any disease process that can affect arteries may also affect the arteries that supply the penis. Men with coronary artery disease (sometimes manifested as **angina**, which is a pain in the chest, with a feeling of suffocation), cerebrovascular disease (which may have caused prior stroke or transient ischemic attack), peripheral vascular disease (decreased blood flow to the legs, often associated with aches/cramps in the legs when attempting to walk for a distance), high blood pressure, and high cholesterol levels are at increased risk for erectile troubles. Men who have experienced severe pelvic or perineal trauma, such as from a motor vehicle accident causing a pelvic fracture or direct injury to the penis, are at risk for erectile dysfunction.

Radiation therapy (administration of radiation to kill cancer cells) to the pelvis for colon cancer or prostate cancer can cause damage to the blood vessels supplying the penis. Erectile dysfunction has been reported in 15% to 65% of men undergoing **external-beam radiation therapy** (EBRT—high-energy radiation beams passed through the skin) for prostate cancer. The onset of erectile dysfunction after radiation therapy is usually not immediate; it typically occurs 2 or more years after the radiation therapy. Interstitial seed therapy for prostate cancer also affects erectile function in 25% to 60% of men who undergo it. As with external-beam radiation therapy, the effect on erectile function is usually seen a year or more after seed placement. Smoking causes **vasospasm,** or tightening up of the arteries, but it also may cause **atherosclerosis,** or **hardening of the arteries.** Venous leaks or abnormal veins may result from prior trauma and may be identified in **Pey-**

Angina

Pain in the chest, with a feeling of suffocation, that occurs with decreased blood flow and oxygenation to the heart.

Radiation therapy

Administration of radiation to treat a disease.

External-beam radiation therapy (EBRT)

A specific radiation technique that is used to treat many types of cancer. Beams of high-energy radiation pass through the skin, with the maximal energy focused on the target organ, e.g., the prostate.

Vasospasm

Constriction of the arteries.

Atherosclerosis

Hardening of the arteries.

ronie's disease, a benign condition affecting the penis in middle-age men (see Questions 31 and 32).

Other Conditions That Cause Erectile Dysfunction

Erectile dysfunction occurs to different degrees in different medical conditions. In men with hypertension, for example, erectile dysfunction occurs in about 27%. The Massachusetts Male Aging Study found an association between low concentration of **high-density lipoproteins** (**HDL**—the "good" cholesterol) and erectile dysfunction, even though there was no correlation between erectile dysfunction and total cholesterol levels. (**Cholesterol** is a fat-like substance that is important to certain body functions but, when present in excessive amounts, contributes to unhealthy fatty deposits in the arteries, which may interfere with blood flow.) In men between the ages of 40 and 55, the risk of moderate erectile dysfunction increased from 6.7% to 25% when the HDL level decreased from 90 to 30 mg/dL. This study also found a similar effect of the HDL level on erectile function in the older male population. Another study *did* find a relationship between the total cholesterol and erectile function; according to this study, the risk of erectile dysfunction increased as total cholesterol level increased. This study also found a negative correlation between HDL level and risk of erectile dysfunction—meaning that the higher the HDL level, the lower the risk of erectile dysfunction. This increased risk of erectile dysfunction with low HDL levels and elevated cholesterol levels is not surprising, because these are the factors that increase one's risk of cardiovascular disease.

Another condition in which erectile dysfunction commonly occurs is **diabetes mellitus**. An estimated 15.7

Hardening of the arteries
Descriptive expression that commonly refers to a group of diseases (forms of arteriosclerosis) characterized by abnormal thickening and hardening (sclerosis) of arterial walls, in which the arteries lose their elasticity. If the thickening/hardening is significant, it may interfere with blood flow.

Peyronie's disease
A benign (noncancerous) condition of the penis that tends to affect middle-aged men. It is characterized by the formation of plaques in the tunica albuginea of the penis and may cause erectile dysfunction.

High-density lipoproteins (HDL)
Often called the "good" cholesterol.

Cholesterol
A fat-like substance important to certain body functions but which, in excessive amounts, contributes to unhealthy fatty deposits in the arteries that may interfere with blood flow.

Diabetes mellitus
A chronic disease associated with high levels of sugar (glucose) in the blood.

million people in the United States have diabetes, including 7.5 million men. Type 2 diabetes, also called **non–insulin-dependent diabetes mellitus**, accounts for 90–95% of the cases of diabetes mellitus; type 1 diabetes, or **insulin-dependent diabetes mellitus**, accounts for 5–10%. The prevalence of erectile dysfunction in diabetes ranges from 35–75%. In men with treated diabetes mellitus in the Massachusetts Male Aging Study, the age-adjusted prevalence of complete erectile dysfunction (no erections at any time) was 28%, which was about three times higher than the prevalence of complete erectile dysfunction in the entire sample of men in the Massachusetts Male Aging Study. The exact cause of erectile dysfunction in men with diabetes mellitus remains to be determined. One possible cause is the presence of certain chemicals associated with diabetes called **glycosylated end-products**, which have been shown to decrease the activity of **nitric oxide** in the body and may also affect the response of blood vessels to nitric oxide. Nitric oxide is important for the production of the neurotransmitter **cGMP**, which causes the relaxation of the smooth muscles in the penis and arteries to allow for increased blood flow into the penis (Figure 4), so anything that adversely affects nitric oxide might also interrupt cGMP production, and thus damage erectile function. There may also be a neurologic component to diabetes mellitus–related erectile dysfunction. The incidence of erectile dysfunction is about 30% lower in type 2 diabetes mellitus than in type 1. In both type 1 and type 2 diabetics, fair or poor metabolic control is associated with an increased risk of erectile dysfunction. The frequency of erectile dysfunction also appears to be related to the duration of diabetes for both type 1 and type 2

Non–insulin-dependent diabetes mellitus

Diabetes that occurs because cells in the body do not respond well to insulin.

Insulin-dependent diabetes mellitus

Diabetes that occurs because the body does not produce sufficient insulin.

Glycosylated end-products

Chemicals associated with diabetes that increase nitric oxide activity in the body.

Nitric oxide

A chemical that affects production of cGMP.

cGMP

A neurotransmitter that causes relaxation of smooth muscles in the penis to permit increased blood flow.

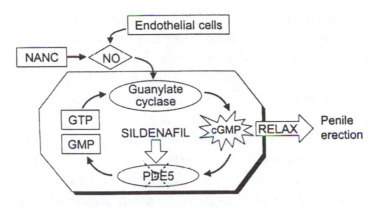

Figure 4   Neurologic mechanism of erectile function. Sexual stimulation leads to release of nitric oxide, which leads to an increase in cGMP, a neurotransmitter that causes smooth muscle relaxation and increased blood flow into the penis. Abbreviations within the figure are: cGMP, cyclic guanosine monophosphate; GMP, guanosine monophosphate; GTP, guanosine triphosphate; NANC, nonadrenergic-noncholinergic neurons; NO, nitric oxide; PDE5, phosphodiesterase type 5. Reprinted with permission from Am J Cardiol 1999; 84(5B): 11N–17N.

diabetics. There is also a positive correlation between the presence of complications of diabetes (neuropathy, vascular diseases, retinopathy, and nephropathy) and the incidence of erectile dysfunction in both type 1 and type 2 diabetics. In type 1 diabetics, the risk of erectile dysfunction was higher in those with a higher body mass index.

Erectile dysfunction occurs in a large number (82%) of men on hemodialysis for renal (kidney) failure. Men on hemodialysis are more likely to experience erectile dysfunction if they are older, if they have diabetes mellitus, and if they do not use medications called angiotensin-converting enzyme (ACE) inhibitors. The cause of the erectile dysfunction is probably multifactorial; it may be partly related to the medical condition that caused the renal failure (e.g., diabetes mellitus), but it also may be related to hormonal changes that occur with dialysis. Dialysis patients have lower testosterone levels and may have high prolactin levels. In addition, dialysis lowers zinc levels and may cause overactivity of the parathyroid gland (hyperparathyroidism).

Smoking may be an independent risk factor for erectile dysfunction, particularly erectile dysfunction caused by vascular disease, and it may also contribute to other causes of erectile dysfunction. In the Massachusetts Male Aging Study, neither the number of cigarettes smoked nor the duration of time smoking had an effect on the incidence of erectile dysfunction. However, the study did show a significant relationship between smoking and erectile dysfunction for certain categories of men. In men who were being treated for heart disease, complete erectile dysfunction was 56% for current smokers, compared with 21% for nonsmokers, after correction for differences in age. Similar results were noted for men with high blood pressure (20% incidence of erectile dysfunction in current smokers versus 8.5% in nonsmokers), those with arthritis (20% in current smokers versus 9.4% in nonsmokers), those taking heart medications (41% in current smokers versus 14% in nonsmokers), and those taking medications for high blood pressure (21% for current smokers versus 7.5% in nonsmokers).

Where alcohol use is concerned, as the saying goes, "Too much of a good thing is bad." Alcohol is thought of as a relaxant, and its use will take away one's inhibitions. Yet alcohol abuse—regular drinking to excess—can cause erectile dysfunction; occasional use does not. Liver failure as a result of alcohol abuse may also affect erectile function.

Purely **psychogenic** (originating from the mind or psyche) erectile dysfunction probably accounts for only 10% of the cases of erectile dysfunction. Depression, anxiety, and stress may have an adverse effect on erectile function, and many of the medications used to treat these problems can cause erectile dysfunction and other forms of sexual dysfunction. However, in most situations, once erectile dysfunction occurs the man develops psychogenic components related to the anxieties that erectile dysfunction causes. Psychogenic causes of erectile dysfunction include

- Performance anxiety
- Depression
- Marital problems
- Dysfunctional attitude toward sex
- Sexual phobia
- Religious beliefs/inhibitions
- Prior traumatic sexual experience

A variety of other medical conditions have been associated with erectile dysfunction, including endocrine abnormalities, such as hyperthyroidism (overactive thyroid gland), hypothyroidism (underactive thyroid gland), **hypogonadism** (when the testes do not produce enough testosterone), and pituitary dysfunction (sometimes manifested by **hyperprolactinemia**, or excess prolactin production).

Medications That Cause Erectile Dysfunction

Hypertension (high blood pressure) may be a risk factor for erectile dysfunction, and several blood pressure medications (antihypertensives) have been described as causing erectile dysfunction, most notably beta-blockers, such as metoprolol, atenolol, and labetolol, and thiazide diuretics such as hydrochlorothiazide.

Psychogenic

Originating from the mind or psyche.

Hypogonadism

A condition in which the testes are not producing adequate testosterone. This may occur because of a testicular problem or because of a lack of stimulation of the testes by the brain.

Hyperprolactinemia

A condition of excess prolactin production. This may be related to a tumor of the pituitary gland but also may be caused by certain medications.

Hypertension

High blood pressure.

The only thiazide diuretic that has not been associated with erectile dysfunction is indapamide. In a study comparing five different blood pressure medications for the treatment of mild hypertension, the highest incidence of erectile dysfunction (17%), was noted in men taking the thiazide diuretic chlorthalidone (Hygroton), and the lowest rate of erectile trouble was noted with the alpha-blocker doxazosin (Cardura). In fact, in this study, some men with pre-existing erectile troubles noted an improvement in erectile function while they were taking doxazosin.

Another group of blood pressure medications, the beta-blockers, have also been associated with erectile dysfunction. The incidence of erectile dysfunction in men taking the beta-blocker propranolol is as high as 15%. Propranolol (Indeval) and other beta-blockers may lower the serum testosterone level to a lesser degree. Clonidine (Catapres), another blood pressure medication, is also associated with an increased incidence of erectile dysfunction.

Antidepressants

Medications to alleviate clinical depression.

Selective serotonin reuptake inhibitors (SSRIs)

Used for depression and also for premature ejaculation.

The incidence of erectile dysfunction in patients taking **antidepressants** has been reported to be as high as 35%. Tricyclic antidepressants, such as imipramine (Tofranil), amitriptyline (Elavil), protriptyline (Concordin), and clomipramine (Anafranil), have been reported to cause erectile dysfunction. It appears that they affect ejaculatory function more than erectile function. **Selective serotonin reuptake inhibitors (SSRIs)** were initially thought to have less of an effect on erectile function; however, studies suggest that 50% of men who are taking SSRIs may experience erectile dysfunction. There have been reports of erectile dysfunction being associated with fluvoxamine (Luvox), fluoxetine (Prozac), sertraline (Zoloft), and paroxetine

(Paxil). In rare cases, erectile dysfunction has *improved* with SSRI use. Antipsychotics such as thioridazine (Mellaril), fluphenazine (Prolixin), and thiothixene (Navane) have also been associated with erectile dysfunction, with up to 44% of men taking thioridazine reporting erectile dysfunction. Benzodiazepines, used to treat such conditions as post-traumatic stress disorder, may also cause erectile dysfunction. Clonazepam (Klonopin) use has been associated with a 43% incidence of erectile dysfunction, whereas the other benzodiazepines and the tranquilizers diazepam (Valium), lorazepam (Ativan), and alprazolam (Xanax) have not been associated with erectile dysfunction.

Cimetidine (Tagamet), a histamine$_2$-antagonist used for gastrointestinal irritation, has been reported to cause erectile dysfunction in 40% of men. It is known to prevent testosterone from functioning and may also increase **prolactin** levels, which can lower testosterone levels, decrease libido, and affect erectile function. The other histamine$_2$-antagonists, ranitidine (Zantac) and famotidine (Pepcid), do not have the same effect on testosterone and are not as frequently associated with erectile dysfunction.

Medications used to lower one's cholesterol (lipid) level may also affect erectile function. Patients taking clofibrate (Atromid-S) often report erectile dysfunction as a **side effect** (a reaction to the treatment). There are also several reports of erectile dysfunction associated with gemfibrozil (Lopid) use and resolution of the erectile dysfunction with discontinuation of the drug. Similarly, the lipid-lowering medications pravastatin (Pravachol) and lovastatin (Mevacor) have also been associated with erectile dysfunction. Digoxin, a cardiac medication, has also been associated with erectile dysfunction,

Prolactin

One of the hormones produced by the pituitary gland. In males, elevated prolactin levels can lower testosterone levels, decrease libido, and affect erectile function.

Side effect

A reaction to a medication or treatment.

as have the seizure medications phenytoin (Dilantin), carbamazepine (Tegretol), primidone (Mysoline), and phenobarbitol (10% to 20% incidence).

Orchiectomy

Removal of the testicle(s).

Hormone therapies for prostate cancer, such as leuprolide (Lupron) and goserelin (Zoladex), **orchiectomy** (removal of the testicles, in this case, to stop most testosterone production), and estrogen, have a negative effect on erectile function. Recreational drugs, including alcohol, cocaine, marijuana, and heroin, may also have a negative effect on erectile function. Up to 50% to 80% of alcoholics experience erectile dysfunction; the erectile dysfunction may resolve with prolonged abstinence, but in some men it may persist. Marijuana decreases testosterone levels, and long-term marijuana use may affect erectile function. Opiate addiction is commonly associated with loss of **libido** (interest in sex) and erectile dysfunction. With abstinence from opiates, the erectile dysfunction improves. Anabolic steroids, used by body builders and athletes to increase their muscle mass, cause testicular atrophy and decrease testosterone production, which may decrease sperm production, decrease libido, and cause erectile dysfunction. If the anabolic steroids are discontinued, it may take 4 months for the testicles to start producing enough testosterone to restore erectile function to normal. The medication ketoconazole, if taken in large quantities, may also affect testosterone production and affect erectile function.

Libido

Sexual desire; one's interest in sex.

5. Is erectile dysfunction or sexual dysfunction a normal process of aging?

Older men often note that it takes longer to achieve an erection; in fact, men over 50 can take 2 to 3 times longer to develop an erection than younger men. The erection may not be as rigid as in younger years, and arousal alone may not lead to full rigidity without tactile (touch) stimulation. It may also take longer to climax. **Ejaculation** (the release of **semen** through the penis during orgasm) may not occur, or it may occur with less force. The recovery period after ejaculation increases with age, and many men over the age of 55 years are not able to have another erection for 12 to 24 hours after ejaculating. *These normal changes related to aging should not be confused with sexual dysfunction or erectile dysfunction;* failure to understand these normal changes and to adapt to them may cause stress and anxiety and may complicate erectile function. In erectile dysfunction, the erections are either inadequate for penetration or do not last long enough for completion of sexual performance. In short, the incidence of erectile dysfunction does increase with age, but it is not an *expected* process of aging.

Age-related changes in sexual function do occur and include a decrease in the amount of smooth muscle in the penis, which may affect erectile function. The sensitivity of the penis can also decrease with age, so that more stimulation is required for an erection. In men over the age of 60, levels of free testosterone in the bloodstream (the active form of testosterone) often decline. Chronic illnesses, which are more common in the elderly, also may decrease testosterone levels, which could affect the vascular response to sexual arousal and libido.

Other factors that are not necessarily restricted to older men can compound age-related changes; for example, morbid obesity and excessive alcohol consumption over a long period of time decrease testosterone levels.

Ejaculation

The release of semen through the penis during orgasm.

Semen

The thick whitish fluid, produced by glands of the male reproductive system, that carries the sperm (reproductive cells) through the penis during ejaculation.

The incidence of erectile dysfunction does increase with age, but it is not an expected *process of aging.*

6. Is erectile dysfunction preventable?

Many medical conditions that can cause erectile dysfunction are inherited, and thus, at this point in time, we cannot prevent them. However, conditions such as hypertension, high cholesterol, and diabetes mellitus can be improved by lifestyle changes, such as exercise and proper diet. If you have diabetes mellitus, tight control of your blood sugar level may not totally prevent the occurrence of erectile dysfunction, but it may prevent the erectile dysfunction from progressing. Avoiding excessive alcohol intake and smoking may also help to decrease your risk of erectile dysfunction. Similarly, if you are a long-distance bicycle rider and experience genital numbness when you finish a bike ride, you may want to start using a bicycle seat designed to put less pressure on the **perineum** (the area under your **scrotum**, the pouch of skin that contains the testicles). New techniques for radical prostatectomy and **investigational** (also called **experimental**, meaning an untested or unproven treatment or approach) techniques, such as nerve grafting at the time of radical prostatectomy, may help decrease the incidence of erectile dysfunction. If you have been diagnosed with prostate cancer and are considering surgery, you may wish to ask your doctor about these procedures.

Perineum

The area under the scrotum.

Scrotum

The pouch of skin that contains the testicles.

Investigational

See *experimental*.

Experimental

An untested or unproven treatment or approach to treatment.

7. Is erectile dysfunction curable?

In most cases, erectile dysfunction is not *curable*—but usually it is *treatable*. The difference is that steps can be taken to help a man have erections—that is what is meant by *treatment*—but these steps cannot reverse the underlying causes of the dysfunction, which is what is meant by *curing* a problem. It is a lot like taking cold medicine: you might feel much better or even normal, but you are still sick with a cold until your body rids itself of the virus on its own. Because most forms of erectile dysfunction are related to underlying diseases, such as hypertension and diabetes—diseases for which there is no cure, merely control—erectile dysfunction is also, in these cases, incurable. However, in select instances, erectile dysfunction is curable. For example, in young, otherwise healthy men who suffer an acute injury to one of the penile arteries that leads to narrowing or blockage of the artery, a surgical procedure may be performed to re-establish blood flow to the penis. **Penile arterial bypass surgery**, similar to arterial bypass surgery performed for blocked blood vessels to the heart or the legs, can be performed for damage to penile arteries. Candidates for penile arterial bypass surgery must have only an arterial cause of their erectile dysfunction. There must be no evidence of any other causes of their erectile dysfunction, such as venous leak, neurologic problems, or hormonal abnormalities. In addition, they should not have any underlying disease processes that would adversely affect the bypass, such as elevated cholesterol, diabetes, and high blood pressure, and they may not smoke (see Questions 71–74).

Similarly, individuals with a pure **venous leak** (i.e., veins that do not compress, allowing blood to drain out of the penis during the erection) who have had radiographic documentation of the leak are candidates for **venous ligation surgery**. In this procedure, the leaky veins are ligated to prevent blood from continually flowing out of the penis during the erection. As with

Penile arterial bypass surgery

A surgical procedure that provides an alternate pathway to bring blood flow into the penis that does not rely on the obstructed artery.

Venous leak

Veins that do not compress to prevent blood from draining out of the corpora during erection. Venous leak may also refer to the rare occasions in which abnormally located veins allow for persistent drainage of blood during an erection.

Venous ligation surgery

A surgical procedure in which leaky veins in the penis are ligated to prevent blood from continually flowing out of the penis during erection.

Urologist

A doctor that specializes in the evaluation and treatment of diseases of the genitourinary tract in men and women.

Genitourinary tract

The urinary system (kidneys, ureters and bladder, and urethra) and the genitalia (in the male, the prostate, seminal vesicles, vas deferens, and testicles).

Prosthesis

An artificial device used to replace the lost normal function of a structure or organ in the body.

Organ

Tissues in the body that work together to perform a specific function (e.g., heart, bladder, penis).

Emission

A discharge, either voluntary or involuntary, of semen from the ejaculatory duct into the urethra.

Detumescence

Subsidence of swelling or turgor; with respect to erections, loss of rigidity.

penile arterial bypass surgery, this surgery requires a skilled **urologist** (a doctor specializing in the evaluation and treatment of diseases of the **genitourinary tract,** consisting of the urinary system and the genitalia, in men and women) who is familiar with this procedure (see Questions 75–78).

Previously potent men who undergo a nerve-sparing radical prostatectomy and experience postoperative erectile dysfunction may experience a return of their erectile function during the first two years after their surgery. Treating the erectile dysfunction early and increasing the penile blood flow may improve erectile function. Finally, men with a psychogenic cause may note resolution of their erectile dysfunction with appropriate treatment of their psychological problems.

Where surgery and psychotherapy are not able to resolve the problem, other treatment methods, such as medical therapy (oral, intraurethral, and intracavernous) and mechanical devices (the vacuum device or a **prosthesis,** i.e., a device used to replace the lost normal function of a structure or **organ**) can help most men achieve a satisfactory erection when desired. These methods are described in Part 4: Treatment.

8. What is sexual dysfunction?

The term *sexual dysfunction* broadly encompasses trouble with any component of the sexual response cycle. The sexual response cycle in men consists of sexual desire/interest, sexual arousal (erection), orgasm (including **emission** [involuntary discharge of semen from the ejaculatory duct into the urethra] and ejaculation), and **detumescence** (return of the penis to the flaccid, non-erect state). An abnormality in one component of the sexual response cycle may not affect the remainder of the components of the cycle. For example, one may still be able to climax and ejaculate without achieving a rigid erection. Common sexual dysfunctions include problems with libido, ejaculation, and orgasm.

Libido

Lack of interest in sex is often called decreased libido or decreased desire. Libido is governed by psychogenic factors and involves all five senses (sight, smell, taste, touch, and hearing) as well as hormonal factors. Low libido, or hypoactive sexual desire, occurs in about 15% of men and in about 20% of the general population, both men and women. Depression and anxiety may adversely affect one's libido, and depression is the leading cause of hypoactive sexual desire. Other causes of hypoactive desire include relationship factors: lack of trust, intimacy conflicts, and lack of physical attraction to one's partner. The hormone **testosterone** is the main hormone responsible for libido in men. Testosterone levels have an effect on libido and on sexual thoughts and fantasies.

Sexual arousal requires input from nerves and arteries. To achieve an adequate erection, there must be at least a six-fold increase in blood flow into the corpora cavernosa. Changes in nerves, arteries, and veins may lead to trouble with erections.

Ejaculation

Ejaculatory dysfunction includes premature ejaculation, retrograde ejaculation, delayed ejaculation, and anejaculation. **Premature ejaculation** means that ejaculation occurs too quickly and may occur with light

Testosterone

The male hormone; it is responsible for secondary sex characteristics, such as hair growth and voice change. It is also the key hormone involved in sexual desire (libido).

Ejaculatory dysfunction

An abnormality of ejaculatory function, such as retrograde ejaculation, premature ejaculation, delayed ejaculation, and anejaculation.

Premature ejaculation

Ejaculation that occurs too quickly.

stimulation before, on, or shortly after penetration, or simply before one wishes for it to occur. **Retrograde ejaculation** is a condition in which the ejaculate passes backward into the bladder; this condition may be associated with decreased ejaculate volume or no ejaculate. **Delayed ejaculation** is a condition in which it takes too long to ejaculate; it is frequently associated with the use of the newer antidepressants, the SSRIs. **Anejaculation** is a condition in which no ejaculation occurs at all. See Table 2 for a list of medications that may affect ejaculation.

Orgasm

Orgasm is another term used for sexual climax, or the culmination of sexual excitement. **Orgasmic dysfunction** refers to alterations in orgasmic function or the inability to achieve an orgasm, to climax. **Anorgasmia** (complete absence of orgasm) occurs in 17% of married men and affects younger men more commonly. Psychological causes of anorgasmia include fear of pregnancy or AIDS, anxiety disorders, and repressive cultural, parental, or religious attitudes toward sexuality.

9. Do women have problems with sexual function?

Yes—in fact, sexual dysfunctions are more common in women than in men (Figure 5). Unlike men, sexual dysfunction tends to affect younger women more commonly than older women, but it is reported across the

---

Retrograde ejaculation

A condition whereby the ejaculate passes backwards into the bladder instead of forward out the tip of the penis; frequently occurs after TURP.

Delayed ejaculation

Taking a longer time to ejaculate, an effect of some antidepressants.

Anejaculation

Inability to ejaculate.

Orgasm

Sexual climax, the culmination of sexual excitement.

Orgasmic dysfunction

Changes in orgasmic function or inability to achieve an orgasm.

Anorgasmia

Failure to experience an orgasm during sex. Congenital anorgasmia is rare and is believed to be related to an overstrict upbringing. Acquired anorgasmia may be caused by medical therapy.

Table 2   Medications That Affect Ejaculation

Medications Associated with Impairment of Ejaculation

Alcohol

Amitriptyline (Elavil, Endep)

Baclofen (Lioresal)

Bethanidine

Chlordiazepoxide (Librium)

Chlorimipramine

Chlorpromazine (Thorazine)

Chlorprothixene (Taractan)

Clomipramine (Anafranil)

Epsilon aminocaproic acid (Amicar)

Guanethidine sulfate (Ismelin)

Haloperidol (Haldol)

Hexamethonium

Imipramine hydrochloride (Tofranil)

Methadone (Dolophine)

Naproxen (Naprosyn)

Pargyline (Eutonyl)

Perphenazine (Etrafon)

Phenelzine sulfate (Nardil)

Phenoxybenzamine hydrochloride (Dibenzyline)

Phentolamine

Prazosin hydrochloride (Minipress)

Reserpine (Serpasil)

SSRIs—selective serotonin reuptake inhibitors: Fluoxetine, paroxetine, sertraline

Thiazides (hydrochlorothiazide)

Thioridazine (Mellaril)

Trifluoroperazine (Stelazine)

(continued)

Table 2 (continued)

Drugs Used to Promote Seminal Emission

Brompheniramine maleate (Bromfed)

Chlorpheniramine (Chlor-Trimeton)

Ephedrine sulfate

Imipramine hydrochloride

Phenylpropanolamine (Entex, Hycomine, Profen)

Pseudoephedrine hydrochloride (Sudafed)

(Adapted from Wang R, Monga M, Hellstrom WJG. Ejaculatory dysfunction. In: Comhaire FH, ed. Male Infertility: Clinical Investigation, Cause, Evaluation and Treatment. London: Chapman and Hall, 1996:205–221.)

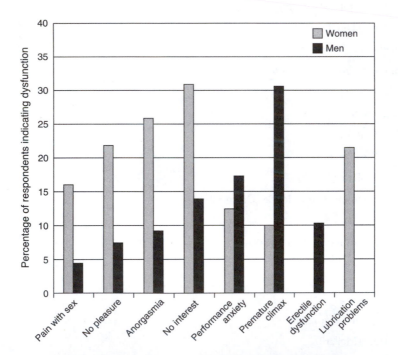

Figure 5   Sexual dysfunction in men and women aged 18 to 59. Adapted with permission from Laumann EO, Gagnon JH, Michael RT, et al. The Social Organization of Sexuality: Sexual Practices in the United States. Chicago, IL: University of Chicago Press, 1994.

life span in women. Just like men, women experience decreased libido/sexual desire, have problems with sexual arousal, or experience pain with intercourse. Decreased sexual desire is the most common female sexual complaint. Problems with the ability to respond to sexual stimulation (vaginal lubrication and swelling response) occur in 14–19% of women. Recent studies have suggested that such problems with female sexual arousal may result from factors similar to those associated with male erectile dysfunction, particularly medical conditions associated with vascular insufficiency. Dyspareunia, recurrent or persistent genital pain in association with sexual intercourse, is common in women and affects 10–15% of women, whereas it rarely affects men.

Just like men, women experience decreased libido/sexual desire, have problems with sexual arousal, or experience pain with intercourse.

Only recently has progress been made in gaining a better understanding of female sexual dysfunction and developing the appropriate tools to evaluate female sexual dysfunction. Future therapies for female sexual dysfunction will depend on such information. Studies have already been performed that assess the response of oral therapy, sildenafil (Viagra), on female sexual dysfunction, and the results of these investigations have demonstrated that Viagra increases female genital blood flow and thus increases vaginal lubrication. Viagra is not, however, approved for use in women by the **U.S. Food and Drug Administration (FDA)**, which is the federal agency responsible for the approval of prescription medication in the United States.

Food and Drug Administration (FDA)

The Food and Drug Administration is responsible for the approval of prescription medications in the United States.

This knowledge may be of little use in treating erectile dysfunction, but it might be a comfort to know that you are not the only one to occasionally have such troubles.

10. What causes decreased libido?

Your interest in sex is governed by **sex hormones** (substances responsible for secondary sex characteristics, e.g., hair growth and voice change in males), primarily testosterone, and by psychosocial factors. Low testosterone levels are associated with decreased libido. Stress, depression, or anxiety may also affect your libido. In men with erectile dysfunction, interest in sex may be diminished as a result of their inability to achieve an adequate erection.

Any man with decreased libido should have his serum testosterone level checked. Normally, there is a "feedback loop" between the brain and the **testes** (two male reproductive organs that are located within the scrotum and produce testosterone and sperm). The brain, through the release of a chemical called **luteinizing hormone (LH),** tells the testicles to produce testosterone. The production of testosterone by the testicles acts on the brain to decrease the release of LH. If the testicles do not produce enough testosterone, the brain releases more LH in an attempt to stimulate the testicles to produce more testosterone. If the brain does not release enough LH, the testicles will not produce enough testosterone. This problem may occur in men with brain tumors or congenital abnormalities.

Another problem that can affect testosterone production is overactivity of the pituitary gland. The **pituitary gland** is a gland in the brain that is composed of two parts, the anterior lobe and the posterior lobe. The anterior lobe produces such hormones as luteinizing hormone and prolactin. Overactivity of the pituitary gland can be caused by a **pituitary adenoma (benign** [noncancerous] tumor of the pituitary gland). This

Sex hormones

Substances responsible for secondary sex characteristics.

Testes

Two male reproductive organs located within the scrotum and produce testosterone and sperm. (Singular: testis)

Luteinizing hormone (LH)

A chemical produced by the brain that stimulates the testes to produce testosterone.

Pituitary gland

A gland in the brain that produces a variety of hormones including luteinizing hormone (LH) and prolactin.

Pituitary adenoma

A benign tumor of the pituitary gland. An adenoma of the anterior pituitary may produce excessive amounts of prolactin.

Benign

A growth that is noncancerous.

abnormality can lead to an elevated prolactin level, which in turn suppresses testosterone production. Abnormalities of the testicles themselves that lead to impaired function of the testes may cause the testosterone levels to be low. Such abnormalities may include a history of testicular torsion, a prior history of undescended testes, prior testicular infections, and other congenital anomalies that affect the testes. Removal of both testes (bilateral orchiectomy) for prostate cancer or (rarely) bilateral testicular cancers causes a significant drop in testosterone level and decreases libido. Men with a single testis usually have adequate testosterone production, provided that the remaining testis is normal.

Testosterone levels do decrease as one ages, but this does not usually cause problems with libido.

PART TWO

Evaluating Erectile Dysfunction: What to Expect

How does one diagnose and evaluate erectile dysfunction?

More . . .

11. How does one diagnose and evaluate erectile dysfunction?

Diagnosis and evaluation of erectile dysfunction require a thorough history, complete physical examination, and possibly some laboratory testing.

The **diagnosis** (identification of the cause or presence of a medical problem or disease) and evaluation of erectile dysfunction require a thorough history, complete physical examination, and possibly some laboratory testing (Figure 6). At first, your doctor will want to establish that the problem truly is erectile dysfunction and not some other form of sexual dysfunction (see Question 8). Your doctor may start the visit out by first paraphrasing the definition of erectile dysfunction—the consistent inability to achieve and/or maintain an erection satisfactory for the completion of sexual performance—to make sure that you are both discussing the same problem. Your doctor will also need a **history**, which will involve asking a number of questions about your medical, social, and sexual background. Some of these questions might be uncomfortable or embarrassing, but you should answer them as honestly as possible because this is probably the most important part of the diagnostic process, allowing the physician to identify common risk factors for both organic (having a physical origin) and psychogenic (originating from the mind or psyche) erectile dysfunction.

12. What questions might the doctor ask me during my initial visit?

Questions such as the following will help evaluate the cause and the magnitude of the erectile dysfunction:

- How long have you been experiencing erectile dysfunction?
- Was the onset abrupt or a slow, progressive deterioration in function?

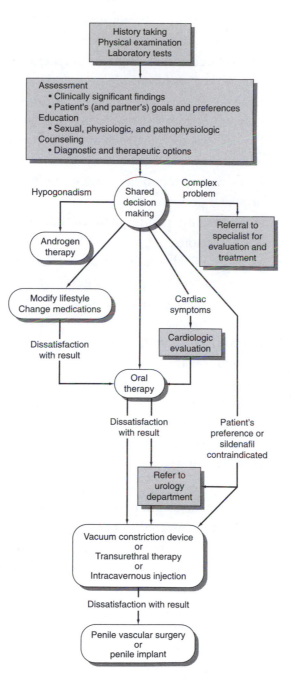

Figure 6   Approach to the evaluation and treatment of erectile dysfunction. Adapted with permission from N Engl J Med 2000;342:1807. Copyright © 2000, The Massachusetts Medical Society.

- Can you identify a precipitating event?
- Is the problem constant or intermittent?
- Does it occur with only one partner or with all partners if there are multiple partners?
- Do you achieve any erection with stimulation, and do you notice nocturnal or evening erections?
- Do you get an erection that is rigid enough for penetration?
- Does your erection last long enough for completion of sexual performance?
- Is there any penile pain or curvature associated with erections?
- What medical conditions do you have?
- Have you had any prior surgery?
- Do you take any medications?
- Do you smoke?
- Do you drink alcohol, and if so, how much?
- Do you use any recreational drugs?
- Do you feel stressed or depressed?
- Is the erectile dysfunction causing you to feel stressed or depressed?
- Is your partner interested in restoring your sexual relationship?

Often, your physician may ask you to complete a questionnaire: the International Index of Erectile Function, or IIEF (see Appendix A, p. 189), an abbreviated questionnaire called the Brief Sexual Function Inventory (BSFI), or the Sexual Health Inventory for Men (SHIM), an abbreviated IIEF that contains five questions (see Appendix B, p. 193). These questionnaires are helpful in assessing your problem and also may help assess your response to therapies.

13. What is the doctor looking for during the physical examination?

The physical examination looks for clinical signs of several disorders including hypertension, cardiovascular disease, renal or liver disease, peripheral vascular disease, thyroid problems, and neurologic problems that may be causing your erectile dysfunction. It is a head-to-toe examination in which your doctor will look at:

- Your heart rate and blood pressure to determine whether there might be a vascular problem.
- Your head and neck to rule out yellow sclera (liver failure) and to check for thyroid enlargement and swollen lymph nodes.
- Your chest to see how well your lungs and heart are working and to look for **gynecomastia** (tender or enlarged breasts in males, which can be a **sign** of a pituitary problem).
- Your **abdomen**, which will be examined by **palpation** (feeling with the hand or fingers, by applying light pressure), to rule out enlarged liver or kidneys, abdominal masses, or tenderness.
- Your **genitalia** (external sexual organs) to make sure that there are no plaques or abnormalities of the penis; the doctor will also check the testes to make sure that both are present, of normal size, and have no tumors and will check secondary sex characteristics, such as pubic hair, that might be responding to lowering of testosterone level.
- Your femoral pulse, located in your thigh, and pulses in your feet to rule out peripheral vascular disease.
- Your penile sensation, reflexes, and rectal tone. This may be uncomfortable: the doctor will check the

Erectile Dysfunction: What to Expect

Gynecomastia

Enlargement or tenderness of the male breast(s).

Sign

Objective evidence of a disease or condition; something that the doctor identifies.

Abdomen

The part of the body below the ribs and above the pelvic bones that contains organs like the intestines, the liver, the kidneys, the stomach, the bladder, and the prostate.

Palpation

Feeling with the hand or fingers, by applying light pressure.

Genitalia

The external sexual organs—in the male the penis, testes, epididymis, and vas deferens.

bulbocavernosus reflex by inserting a finger in your rectum, squeezing the tip of penis, and noting a contraction of the anus at time of squeezing penis. If this reflex is not present, it could indicate that a problem exists in the nerves of the penis.

14. Why is my doctor checking my testosterone level?

There are several reasons why your doctor will check a testosterone level during your initial evaluation. First, he or she can use the results to decide where the underlying problem might lie. For instance, rare benign pituitary tumors can lower testosterone production and cause decreased libido and erectile dysfunction. These tumors are treatable, and the sexual side effects are potentially reversible. Second, the doctor is attempting to determine whether supplemental testosterone can improve poor libido, which might be complicating erectile dysfunction. There is no other way of assessing your testosterone level besides the blood test, because neither libido nor testis size is a good gauge of testosterone levels. Clearly, if you have a decrease in your libido and your testosterone level is low, then supplemental testosterone will enhance your libido, but it might not resolve the erectile dysfunction if there is more going on than simply a low testosterone level. However, there are other theoretical benefits to testosterone supplementation for a low testosterone level (see Question 16). Thus, one of the first steps in evaluating erectile dysfunction is to determine the patient's testosterone level.

15. What effects does testosterone have on my erections?

If you have erectile dysfunction and a normal testosterone level, then giving you additional testosterone will have no significant effect on your libido (your interest is sex) or your erections. If you have erectile dysfunction and a low testosterone level, giving you supplemental testosterone alone will most likely not have a significant effect on your erectile function. Whether or not it makes the penile tissues more sensitive to the therapies for erectile dysfunction, such that you are more likely to respond to therapy, is unclear. Therefore, your doctor will not routinely give testosterone supplementation solely to enhance erectile function. As noted in the following questions, there are other benefits to testosterone therapy that you may find worthwhile after considering the potential risks.

16. How else does the testosterone level affect me?

It is becoming increasingly apparent that testosterone has other functions besides its effect on libido. Testosterone or testosterone derivatives appear to be important in maintaining bone density, thereby preventing osteoporosis. Testosterone may also have an effect on lean body mass, **red blood cell** count (red blood cells carry oxygen to the tissues), and general sense of well being. Thus, there are other theoretical benefits to hormonal therapy.

Red blood cells

The cells in the blood that carry oxygen to the tissues.

17. What happens after the history, physical examination, and laboratory tests have been carried out?

In most cases, once possible causes have been identified and evaluated, your doctor may discuss lifestyle changes and possible therapies with you. This goal-oriented approach centers around the doctor and patient discussing possible origins of the problem and then making a decision about therapy (Figure 6). In select cases, when the patient wants to know more about the cause of the erectile dysfunction—is it really an artery problem or a vein problem?—then further investigation is required. Young men with no identifiable medical conditions or risk factors should undergo further evaluation because these individuals are the best candidates for penile vascular surgery.

If there appears to be a significant psychological component to the erectile dysfunction, then it may be appropriate to seek consultation with a psychiatrist, psychologist, or sex therapist. Although organic problems account for 80% to 90% of the cases of erectile dysfunction, realistically, in many men there is some psychological overlay. Treating the erectile dysfunction may resolve psychological problems related to erectile dysfunction, but if there are significant psychological stressors, then psychological counseling at the same time as medical therapy may be more beneficial than medical therapy alone.

It is important to identify possible causes of your erectile dysfunction so that you and your doctor can find the best method of treating it.

It is important to identify possible causes of your erectile dysfunction so that you and your doctor can find the best method of treating it. The success rates of many therapies have been subdivided based on the causes and the degree of erectile dysfunction. Knowing where your problem comes from will allow you to determine the likelihood of success of a given therapy and to avoid falsely elevated expectations.

It is often very helpful if your partner can participate in the evaluation and treatment process. Realistically, an intervention is unlikely to succeed if your partner is not interested in resuming sexual relations. For example, if your partner is a postmenopausal woman, she might suffer from a condition that is common in postmenopausal women called atrophic vaginitis, which stems from lower estrogen levels that cause the vaginal mucosa to become thin, dry, and prone to irritation. If this is the case, she may find intercourse uncomfortable—and you may not have a supportive partner to help you through the therapy for your erectile dysfunction. This might be an opportunity to address both problems; discomfort from atrophic vaginitis can be improved by using lubricants during intercourse. In addition, the use of topical estrogen cream helps restore the vaginal mucosa in women for whom such agents are appropriate, so your partner may want to discuss with her primary care provider or gynecologist the risks and benefits of topical estrogen therapy for atrophic vaginitis.

18. What laboratory tests are performed?

The laboratory evaluation of erectile dysfunction is limited in most cases. If you are treated by a primary care provider on a regular basis, such information as a fasting blood sugar, kidney function tests, liver function tests, and lipid profile are often available. If you have experienced unexplainable weight gain or loss and/or other signs or symptoms of abnormal thyroid function, then thyroid function tests may be performed. All men with erectile dysfunction should have a serum testosterone level checked. Because the testosterone level varies throughout the day and tends to be highest in the morning, it is best to have the testosterone level checked in the morning. In some men, such as obese men and those with liver disease, the total testosterone level may be low, but the free testosterone level (the active form of testosterone) is normal. If the testosterone level is low, then a prolactin level should be checked to rule out a pituitary adenoma (a benign brain tumor).

19. Do I need any specialized tests?

In most cases, the history, physical examination, and blood testing allow the physician to identify possible causes of your erectile dysfunction, but in some cases, a more advanced evaluation may be required. In men who seem to have a psychogenic basis for their problem, the doctor might order **nocturnal penile tumescence (NPT) studies** to confirm this theory (see Question 20). (**Tumescence** is the state of being swollen, in this case referring to penile rigidity.) This test involves wearing a specialized device around the penis at night on several occasions when one goes to sleep. The device records whether you have erections during your sleep, which is both normal and common; if you do, it would suggest that the erectile dysfunction could be psychogenic in origin, which can help determine the correct treatment strategy. However, NPT studies have limitations (see Question 20), and it has been suggested that sleep-related erections may not be the same as sexually induced erections.

Nocturnal penile tumescence (NPT) study

A specialized study that evaluates the frequency and the quality of nocturnal erections.

Tumescence

Condition of being tumid or swollen; with respect to erections, penile rigidity.

If your doctor wishes to evaluate your penile vasculature and obtain a preliminary assessment of the arterial and venous function therein, the best initial test is **Doppler ultrasonography** (use of a Doppler probe during ultrasound to look at flow through vessels) in conjunction with injection therapy. In **ultrasound** studies, internal organs are visualized by measurement of reflected sound waves. In this particular study, you are injected with a chemical that causes smooth muscle relaxation and increases penile blood flow, usually 10 µg of alprostadil (Caverject), but other agents, such as trimix/triple P (prostaglandin E_1, papaverine, and phentolamine), may be used. After injection, sequential blood flow studies are performed. The rate at which blood is flowing through the cavernosal artery on each side of the penis (the peak systolic velocity) can be determined. A peak systolic velocity over 25 to 30 mL/sec is considered normal. The Doppler ultrasound also allows the diameter of the cavernosal arteries to be measured. In addition, the function of the penile veins can be assessed by measuring the end-diastolic velocity (venous **resistance**). This test may also be affected by patient anxiety and may require stimulation to achieve the maximum response. As with injection therapy, there is a small risk of priapism and penile pain related to the injection or to the medication used. If the Doppler ultrasound study demonstrates an abnormality of the arteries or veins and the patient wishes to be evaluated for possible surgical correction, then further studies would be required. **Arteriography** (see Question 25), the injection of contrast into the arteries that supply the penis to identify areas of narrowing, or **cavernosography** (see Question 24), the injection of contrast into the corpora of the penis and measurements of the pressure within the corpora

Doppler ultrasonography

Use of a Doppler probe during ultrasound to look at flow through vessels.

Ultrasound

A technique used to look at internal organs by measuring reflected sound waves.

Resistance

Opposition to blood flow out of the penis.

Arteriography

A technique employed to identify areas of narrowing in the arteries.

Cavernosography

A technique employed to visualize areas of venous leak.

cavernosa to identify sites of venous leak, are performed to better assess possible arterial or venous abnormalities. These more invasive tests are not required in all individuals and should be performed in select institutions where penile artery bypass surgery or venous ligation surgery is performed.

20. What are nocturnal penile tumescence studies?

Historically, one of the first tests used to evaluate nocturnal penile tumescence was the postage stamp test. With the postage stamp test, one would purchase a roll of stamps and place the stamps snugly around the penis and then go to sleep. The feeling was that if the postage stamps were "popped off" the penis during the night, an adequate erection had occurred. Needless to say, this test did not take into account such factors as restlessness at night, the actual degree of rigidity, and the duration of the rigidity. The Snap-Gauge test was a modification of the postage stamp test. The Snap-Gauge is a Velcro band that was fitted around the penis and had three colored plastic film elements arranged in parallel. Each film ruptured at a radial force selected to correspond to intracavernosal pressures found in erections (90–180 mmHg). Ten ounces of radial force ruptured the blue film, 15 ounces of radial force ruptured the red film, and 20 ounces of radial force ruptured the clear film. The device was worn for three consecutive nights. Although the Snap-Gauge provided more information and was more accurate than the postage stamp test, it still tended to misclassify about one third of patients with erectile dysfunction, and it still could not determine the duration of the rigidity. Formal nocturnal penile tumescence (NPT) testing requires spending two to three consecutive nights in the sleep laboratory. Men undergoing NPT tests must abstain from alcohol, caffeine, and medications that may affect sleep or erections for 8 hours before the test. Because sleep erections occur primarily during **rapid eye movement (REM)** sleep, one must assess the quality of REM sleep, which is done through the use of an electroencephalographic test, an electro-oculographic test, and a submental electromyographic test. To assess penile tumescence, two mercury-in-rubber strain gauges (expandable rubber loops) are placed on the penis, one at the base and the other just behind the glans penis. When the loop circumferences increase, the mercury column is thinned, which increases the electrical resistance through the mercury. Each time there is an increase in the electrical resistance, it is recorded on a tracing. The high point of the deflection on the tracing corresponds to the change in penile circumference. The study also allows one to detect discrepancies between the changes in both loops, meaning that if one loop expands substantially more than the other, the test can detect this. One of the biggest drawbacks of NPTs is that they are measuring nocturnal erections, not erections related to sexual arousal, and each may occur via different mechanisms. Secondly, there can be false-positive NPT results; these more commonly occur in patients with neurogenic erectile dysfunction and pelvic steal syndrome, and false-negative NPT results occur in patients with depression, alcohol use, medication ingestion, and sleep apnea, a condition in which a person stops breathing for a short period of time during sleep (anywhere from a few seconds to a minute or two), causing him to wake repeatedly and get insufficient sleep. In addition, the measurements of penile rigidity with NPT studies may be insufficient to differentiate between organic and psychogenic erectile dysfunction.

Rapid eye movement (REM)

A phase in the sleep cycle. Nocturnal erections occur during this phase of sleep.

Formal nocturnal penile tumescence testing is also laborious and expensive.

21. What is the RigiScan?

The RigiScan (Timm Medical Technologies, Eden Prairie, MN) was developed as a portable home device to evaluate the quality and the quantity of nocturnal penile erections. It is used to provide continuous measurements of penile rigidity and tumescence, and it represents an improvement over previous techniques of assessing nocturnal penile tumescence. The RigiScan consists of a portable battery-powered unit that is strapped around the thigh and has two loops that are connected to a direct-current torque motor. One loop is placed around the base of the penis and the other is placed just below the **corona** (the area of the penis just before the glans penis). To measure tumescence every 30 seconds, the loops tighten and the penile circumference (loop length) is recorded. Fifteen seconds later, a second measurement is taken without active tightening of the loops. If tumescence (measured by the length of the loop) increases by 10 mm or more from the initial measurements, rigidity measurements are taken. Rigidity is measured every 30 seconds by a slight tightening of the loops. Rigidity is expressed as a percentage, with 100% equaling the rigidity of a noncompressible rubber shaft. Rigidity measurements are discontinued when tumescence decreases to within 10 mm of baseline. The RigiScan can record three uninterrupted 10-hour sessions. The information stored in the device can then be downloaded into a microprocessor, and the nocturnal penile tumescence and rigidity information can be analyzed, displayed, and printed. The RigiScan measures only **radial rigidity**, that is, rigidity across the width or circumference; it does not measure **axial**

Corona

The area of the penis just before the glans penis.

Radial rigidity

Rigidity across the width or circumference.

rigidity, or rigidity across the length of the penis. Axial rigidity is the most important measurement in predicting vaginal penetration because it is used to assess the ability of the penis to stay straight despite pressure against the tip.

In most patients, the RigiScan device can distinguish functional from inadequate erections and is helpful in distinguishing psychogenic from organic erectile dysfunction.

Axial rigidity
Rigidity across the length.

22. What is penile Doppler ultrasonography?

This test is usually performed in conjunction with an injection of Caverject/Edex or triple P to increase the flow of blood into the penis. Penile Doppler ultrasonography is a **noninvasive** way (i.e., it does not require an incision or insertion of an instrument or substance into the body) to assess the corpora cavernosa and the functional status of the penile arteries and veins. The use of Doppler allows the blood flow through the arteries to be measured. Normally, cavernosal arterial flow increases to over 25 to 30 mL/sec in response to injection therapy; thus, arterial flow that is less than 25 to 30 mL/sec suggests the presence of arterial disease.

Noninvasive
Not requiring any incision or insertion of an instrument or substance into the body.

The status of the veins is assessed indirectly. When there is no arterial disease and there is adequate inflow, the veins should be compressed against the tunica (the thick white membrane wrapped around the corpora cavernosa), which should prevent blood from flowing out of the veins. If blood flow persists when the veins are compressed, a venous leak may be present.

The study may be performed in the urologist's office, or it may be performed in the radiology department.

The study begins with injection of the Caverject/Edex or triple P. The cavernosal artery on each side of the penis is identified, and the Doppler probe is placed on top of the penis to measure the rate of blood flow through each of the cavernosal arteries to be measured. Sequential measurements are taken every 5 minutes for 15 to 30 minutes. Similarly, venous **resistance** (the amount of opposition to blood flow out of the penis) is calculated and used as a gauge of the status of venous **occlusion** (blockage of flow). If the arterial response is marginal but the patient seems anxious—anxiety sometimes causes constriction of the blood vessels, which decreases the blood flow into the penis—the physician may ask the patient to stimulate himself so that the blood flows can be reassessed, or may inject the patient with additional medication.

An abnormal Doppler study result suggests that vascular disease is the cause of the erectile dysfunction. False-positive results, a study suggesting that vascular disease is present when it is not, may occur if the patient is overly anxious about the study. If the Doppler ultrasound results are positive for vascular disease and the patient is a candidate for vascular surgery, then further investigation with more invasive vascular studies would be required (see Questions 23–25).

23. What is cavernosometry?

Cavernosometry is a specialized erectile dysfunction test that is performed to determine whether there is veno-occlusive dysfunction, that is, whether a vein or veins fail to occlude, allowing blood to continuously drain out of the penis during an erection (venous leak; see Question 7), causing erectile dysfunction. This test is performed by first injecting either 10 µg of alprostadil

Resistance

Opposition to blood flow out of the penis.

Occlusion

Blockage of flow.

Cavernosometry

A somewhat invasive technique used to determine whether a venous leak is present.

(Caverject or Edex) or an equivalent amount of triple P and then placing a small needle that has tubing attached to it (a **butterfly needle**) into each side of the penis into the corpora cavernosa, one for saline infusion and one for pressure monitoring. The rate of infusion that is required to initiate and maintain an erection is noted. An inability to produce a fully rigid erection or to increase the **intracavernous pressure** (pressure within the corpora cavernosa) to 90 mmHg or higher despite an increase in the rate of infusion to 300 mL/minute is indicative of a venous leak. Similarly, a rapid decrease in pressure in the corpora cavernosa after the infusion is stopped is also indicative of venous leak. This test is not routinely performed in all men with a suspected venous leak; rather, it is performed in select individuals who are suspected to have a venous leak and who wish to pursue possible surgical repair.

Butterfly needle

A small needle that has tubing attached to it.

Intracavernous pressure

The pressure within the corpora cavernosa, as measured during cavernosography.

24. What is cavernosography?

Cavernosography is also used in individuals with erectile dysfunction who are suspected of having a venous leak and are interested in pursuing a surgical repair. Similar to cavernosometry, one is first injected with 10 μg of alprostadil or a similar dose of trimix. A butterfly needle is placed into the corpora. In lieu of saline, a contrast material is infused, and **x-ray** studies are obtained periodically during the infusion to allow viewing of the sites of venous leakage for possible subsequent venous ligation procedures.

X-ray

A type of high-energy radiation that can be used at low levels to make images of the internal structure of the body and at high levels for radiation therapy.

25. What is penile arteriography?

Penile arteriography performed with an injected agent that stimulates blood flow, such as Caverject, Edex, or triple P, is considered to be the gold standard test in the identification and localization of arterial disease. Typically, a pharmacologic Doppler ultrasound—meaning an ultrasound performed after use of one of the agents mentioned above—has been obtained before the study and has demonstrated arterial inflow problems. If arterial disease is identified on the Doppler ultrasound study, and the man is a candidate for penile bypass surgery and is interested in being evaluated for the surgery, then pharmacologic penile arteriography would be performed. In reality, this is only a handful of individuals. The best candidate for penile bypass surgery is a young healthy man with a prior history of trauma causing the erectile dysfunction.

Penile arteriography should be performed only at institutions that have experience performing the study because it is one of the most challenging vascular studies to perform. The procedure is performed under **local anesthesia** (anesthesia that is confined to the area being operated on). A dose of Caverject or triple P is injected into the side of the penis at the start of the study to maximize blood flow to the penis and to enhance the yield of the study. The **groin** (area between the lower abdomen and thigh) is anesthetized with a local anesthetic, and then a needle is placed into the femoral artery, the artery in the groin. A small **catheter** (a hollow tube that allows for fluid drainage from or injection into an area) is then passed through the needle and advanced until it is in a good location for injection of the contrast, which allows for x-ray visualization of the arteries. If the patient is very anxious, the study can be difficult to perform because anxiety or stress can cause the arteries to narrow (constrict), making interpretation of the results more difficult. The radiologist performing the study and

Local anesthesia

Anesthesia confined to one part of the body.

Groin

The area between the lower abdomen and the thigh.

Catheter

A hollow tube that allows for fluid drainage from or injection into an area.

your surgeon will review the films to determine whether there are narrowed areas of the artery(ies) that could be responsible for the erectile dysfunction.

PART THREE

What Are the Other Types of Sexual Dysfunction?

What is premature ejaculation?

What is retrograde ejaculation and what causes it?

More ...

26. What is premature ejaculation?

Premature ejaculation is when ejaculation occurs too quickly, such as before penetration or just after penetration. This condition tends to occur more frequently in younger men. Premature ejaculation is the most common form of sexual dysfunction, occurring in 30% to 40% of adult men. The condition may be lifelong or acquired. Despite its prevalence, men rarely seek help for premature ejaculation. There are three criteria for a diagnosis of premature ejaculation:

1. There must be persistent or recurrent ejaculation with minimal stimulation before, on, or shortly after penetration and before the individual wishes it.
2. This must cause marked distress or interpersonal difficulty.
3. The premature ejaculation is not a result of a substance, such as an effect from withdrawal of opioids.

It appears that men with premature ejaculation may have an increased sensitivity and excitability of the glans penis and the dorsal nerve, which supplies sensation to the penis.

Retrograde ejaculation is very common in men who have undergone a transurethral prostatectomy.

27. What is retrograde ejaculation and what causes it?

Retrograde ejaculation occurs when the ejaculate flows backward into the bladder instead of forward and out the tip of the penis. Retrograde ejaculation is very common in men who have underdone a **transurethral prostatectomy (TURP)**, a surgical technique using a specialized instrument that allows the surgeon to remove the prostatic tissue that is bulging into the ure-

Transurethral prostatectomy (TURP)

A surgical procedure to remove prostatic tissue blocking the urethra.

thra and blocking the flow of urine through the urethra. A TURP is usually performed to treat benign enlargement of the **prostate**. Retrograde ejaculation may also occur in men with diabetes mellitus, and sometimes is a side effect of certain medications, including the blood pressure medications phenoxybenzamine (Dibenzyline), phentolamine, prazosin (Minipress), and tamsulosin (Flomax) and the antipsychotic medications thioridazine (Mellaril), chlorpromazine (Thorazine), triflupromazine (Vespein), and mesoridazine (Serentil). In men who have undergone surgery on the bladder neck (bladder outlet), the bladder neck may not close completely, thus allowing the semen to pass backwards into the bladder. Retrograde ejaculation does not cause any harm—one simply urinates out the ejaculate.

Prostate

A gland that surrounds the urethra and is located just under the bladder. It produces fluid that is part of the ejaculate (semen). This fluid provides some nutrient to the sperm.

28. What is anejaculation and what causes it?

Anejaculation is the condition in which there is no flow of ejaculate in either direction. This condition occurs in some men with spinal cord injuries and in some men with cancer of the testis who have undergone surgery to remove affected lymph nodes, a procedure called **retroperitoneal lymph node dissection**. Anejaculation may also occur if the outflow of the ejaculate is blocked; this may be caused by a small stone in the **ejaculatory duct** (the structure through which the ejaculate passes into the urethra), or by prior infection and scarring of the male reproductive tract from sexually transmitted diseases, such as gonorrhea, and other diseases that affect the genitourinary tract, including tuberculosis. In such cases, the ejaculatory duct may be opened surgically. Anejaculation occurs after a radical prostatectomy because the seminal vesicals and

Retroperitoneal lymph node dissection

A procedure to remove lymph nodes adjacent to the site of testicular or prostate cancer.

Ejaculatory duct

The structure through which the ejaculate passes into the urethra.

prostate gland are removed and the **vas deferens**, the tube that sperm passes through to reach the urethra, is tied off. Congenital disorders and their treatment may also cause anejaculation; such treatments include imperforate anus, a condition in which the rectum does not open to the perineal skin, and thus there is no way for stool to exit the body.

29. What is anorgasmia and what causes it?

Anorgasmia, the inability to achieve an orgasm, may be "congenital" or "acquired." **Congenital anorgasmia** is rare and is believed to be related to an overstrict upbringing. Nocturnal emissions ("wet dreams") may occur, but repression of the normal sexual responses prevents the individual from achieving climax and ejaculation. **Acquired anorgasmia** may be caused by medical therapy.

30. What is priapism and prolonged erection?

Priapism is a persistent abnormal erection of the penis, usually without sexual desire, and is accompanied by pain and tenderness. A lack of detumescence is referred to as a **prolonged erection** if the duration of the rigidity is less than 4–6 hours and *priapism* if the erection lasts longer than 4–6 hours. If the erection lasts longer than 6–8 hours, it is often associated with pain. Priapism may occur from too much blood flow into the penis (high flow), or it may be a result of too little blood flow out of the penis (low flow). High-flow priapism may occur after there has been an injury to the penis that causes damage to an artery that results in unregulated blood flow into the penis. Because there is an increase in arterial blood (which carries oxygen) into the penis, high-flow priapism does not cause pain. In high-flow priapism, there is venous drainage out of the penis, so the erection does not tend to be as rigid as in a full erection. Low-flow priapism occurs more in men with **sickle cell disease/trait**—a condition in which the red blood cells take on an abnormal (sickle) shape in response to decreased oxygenation, dehydration, and acidosis—and cancers of the blood, such as **leukemia**. It may also occur with injection therapy for erectile dysfunction (see Question 59) and with certain psychiatric medications, such as trazodone. Because the problem consists of a problem with drainage of blood from the penis, which has little oxygen in it, this form of priapism is associated with pain and full rigidity.

31. What is Peyronie's disease and what causes it?

Peyronie's disease is a benign (noncancerous) condition of the penis that tends to affect middle age males. The incidence is 4.3 per 100,000 men aged 20–29 years and increases to 66 per 100,000 men aged 50–59 years. Approximately two thirds of affected men are between the ages of 40 and 60 years. The exact cause of Peyronie's disease is not known. The disease is characterized by the formation of plaques in the tunica albuginea of the penis. These plaques may be felt on penile examination and at times can feel as hard as bone. The plaques are like scar tissue and affect the function of the tunica in that area. Because the plaque is not elastic and stretchy like the rest of the tunica, it pulls the penis to the side of the plaque during an erection and may also cause "wasting" (an indentation in

Sickle cell disease/sickle cell trait

A condition in which the red blood cells take on an abnormal shape (sickle) in response to decreased oxygenation, dehydration, and acidosis. This abnormal shape makes it difficult for the red blood cells to pass through the blood vessels and leads to blockages of the vessels, causing pain and ischemia to tissues. In the penis, it may lead to priapism.

Leukemia

A cancer of the blood-forming organs that affects the blood cells.

Peyronie's disease is a benign (noncancerous) condition of the penis that tends to affect middle age males.

the penis) at the site of the plaque. There may also be pain associated with an erection. Lastly, because the plaque does not behave like normal tunica, it may also cause erectile troubles. The plaque may occur anywhere along the penile shaft but is more commonly identified on the top (dorsal) surface of the penis. More than one plaque may be palpable. The hallmarks of Peyronie's disease are a palpable plaque (a hard spot along the shaft of the penis that one can feel when examining the penis), penile curvature, and a painful erection.

The disease typically has a slow onset, and most men cannot identify a precipitating factor. Several theories exist as to the cause of Peyronie's disease; the most commonly accepted theory is that minor trauma during intercourse leads to minor tears in the tunica or rupture of small blood vessels. Bleeding and abnormal healing occurs after this injury and produces the plaque. In some men, there is a family history of Peyronie's disease, and 16–20% of men with Peyronie's have a disease called Dupuytren's contractures. Dupuytren's contractures is an inherited condition that causes contractures in the hands that pull the affected fingers inward. An increased incidence of arterial disease (30%) and diabetes with its associated small arterial disease (2.7–12%) has also been noted in men with Peyronie's disease.

The natural history of Peyronie's disease is variable. The disease is thought to have two phases: the acute phase, which usually lasts up to 18 months and is associated with pain, penile curvature, and plaque formation, and a more chronic phase, in which there is minimal or no pain, a palpable plaque, and residual penile curvature. Over time, the disease may progress in about 42% of men, improve in 13%, and remain the same in about 45%. In many cases, the disease produces few symptoms, the curvature does not prevent sexual performance, and there is no pain or associated erectile dysfunction. In such cases, reassurance that there is nothing bad going on is often all that is necessary.

32. How does one evaluate Peyronie's disease?

As with any initial presentation, the evaluation of Peyronie's disease starts with a history of symptoms: duration and presence of pain; current erectile status and erectile status before the onset of the Peyronie's disease; whether symptoms are stable, progressing, or regressing; and degree of penile curvature and its effect on sexual function. The physician will ask about a history of prior penile trauma or manipulation.

Because the penile abnormality has a classic presentation and most men are able to accurately describe the symptoms, little investigation is needed initially. After the history is elicited, an examination will be performed. Examination of the hands will be performed to look for Dupuytren's contractures. Examination of the penis includes assessment of penile length and girth and palpation for penile plaques. In most cases, the physician will ask the man to bring in either a Polaroid photograph or digital picture of his erect penis to demonstrate the degree and the location of the curvature. If the patient is unable to obtain a photograph, the physician may induce an erection in the office by injecting a chemical that causes an erection in order to allow the physician to locate the area of curvature and to assess the degree of curvature. If the man

has erectile dysfunction in addition to the penile curvature, further studies are needed to assess the cause of
the erectile dysfunction.

Erectile dysfunction is found in about 19% of men
with Peyronie's disease. The erectile dysfunction in
Peyronie's disease may be the result of (1) performance
anxiety; (2) the penile deformity preventing intercourse; (3) a flail penis, whereby extensive Peyronie's
disease causes scarring in a segment of the penis that
therefore does not become rigid, while the remainder
is able to become rigid; and (4) an impaired erection,
which may be related to concomitant arterial disease
(36%) or veno-occlusive disease (59%). The use of
penile Doppler ultrasonography with injection of a
dilating agent, such as alprostadil or triple P (see
Question 22) is helpful in determining the cause of the
erectile dysfunction.

PART FOUR

Treatment

What are the current treatment options
for erectile dysfunction?

My testosterone level is low. Should I
receive supplemental testosterone?

What are the benefits and risks
of testosterone therapy?

More . . .

33. What are the current treatment options for erectile dysfunction?

In many societies and cultures, sexual function and problems with sexual function are rarely discussed openly. As a result, research into the pathophysiology and treatment of erectile dysfunction has progressed more slowly than research in many other fields of medicine. The advent of **oral** therapy and the media coverage of Viagra as the first effective oral treatment for erectile dysfunction make us think that there is a heightened awareness and a willingness to discuss erectile dysfunction more openly. This perception is not entirely accurate, however: Before the advent of oral therapy, only some 10% of men with erectile therapy sought help; with the advent of oral therapy, approximately 20% are seeking help.

Because erectile dysfunction is not a disease in and of itself, but rather a manifestation of an underlying disease process, it is important to search for these disease processes during the history and physical examination. Many of these diseases—such as diabetes mellitus, high cholesterol level, and cardiovascular disease—are associated with significant **morbidity** (i.e., illness or disease) and possibly **mortality** (death). Furthermore, erectile dysfunction has been shown to have a significant impact on **quality of life** (an evaluation of healthy status relative to the patient's age, expectations, and physical and mental capabilities), self-esteem, incidence of depression, and partner relationships. Thus the treatment of erectile dysfunction and the underlying causative disease processes may have a significant influence on the overall well-being of the man and affect his partner as well.

Oral

Taken by mouth.

Morbidity

Diseased condition or state.

Mortality

Death in a population at risk.

Quality of life

An evaluation of healthy status relative to the patient's age, expectations, and physical and mental capabilities.

The selection of the appropriate therapy for each individual depends on several factors, including medical, personal, cultural, ethnic, religious, and financial considerations. Each form of therapy has its own advantages and disadvantages that make it more or less suitable for individual patients. Potentially modifiable **risk** factors include the following:

- Lifestyle changes: weight loss, smoking cessation, decrease in alcohol consumption, dietary changes to decrease cholesterol level, avoidance of recreational drugs, and changing one's bicycle seat (if appropriate).

- Improving psychosocial factors: attempting to resolve conflicts with one's partner (if present), stress reduction, and treatment for anxiety or depression (if present).

- Improving one's understanding of sexual function: understanding the **sexual response cycle,** age-related changes in sexual function, and the effects of erectile dysfunction on sexual function.

- Identification of **iatrogenic** causes (i.e., those resulting from treatment, such as surgery, medication, or procedures) of erectile dysfunction. Erectile dysfunction may be the result of certain medications, and in some cases, different medications may be employed.

Most men with erectile dysfunction will not be able to permanently restore their erectile function. Some men who have identifiable vascular causes and no other underlying medical conditions and who are willing to undergo surgery may be candidates for penile arterial

Risk

The chance or probability that a particular event will or will not happen.

Sexual response cycle

The cycle of interest, arousal, climax, ejaculation, and detumescence.

Iatrogenic

Resulting from treatment by a physician, such as from medications, procedures, or surgery.

Treatment

Vacuum device

A device that is used to provide an erection. It consists of three parts: a cylinder, a pump, and a constricting band. The band is preloaded on the bottom of the cylinder, and the cylinder is placed over the penis. The pump, which is connected to the cylinder, creates a suction that pulls blood into the penis. Because the constricting band is placed at the base of the penis, the blood remains in the penis until the band is removed.

Penile prosthesis

A device that is surgically placed into the penis that allows a man with erectile dysfunction to have an erection.

Psychogenic

Stemming from the mind or psyche.

Sildenafil (Viagra)

The first effective, FDA-approved oral therapy for erectile dysfunction. Sildenafil is a phosphodiesterase type 5 inhibitor.

bypass surgery or venous ligation surgery (see Question 71); however, this group includes only a small number of men. Most men require a pill, injection therapy, the **vacuum device,** or a **penile prosthesis** to allow them to achieve an erection when they wish to do so. It is important for your physician to discuss each of these therapies with you, reviewing each option's pros and cons so that you may decide which form of therapy is most appropriate for you and your partner. If the cause of your erectile dysfunction is believed to be **psychogenic** (originating from the mind or psyche), then sexual counseling would be a first-line therapy. It is important to realize that psychosocial factors are important in all forms of erectile dysfunction, and psychosexual therapy may be of benefit to couples with organic erectile dysfunction as well as those with psychogenic erectile dysfunction.

The following therapies are currently available for the treatment of erectile dysfunction:

- Oral therapy: Drugs available in pill form include **sildenafil** (Pfizer's **Viagra**), **vardenafil** (Bayer's **Levitra**), and **tadalafil** (Lily Icos's **Cialis**). Additional oral therapies are under investigation.

- Injection therapy: **Caverject** and **Edex** (both **prostaglandin E$_1$**) are the two FDA-approved therapies; triple P (phentolamine, prostaglandin, and papaverine), papaverine, and bimix (papaverine and phentolamine) are available at certain institutions.

- Mechanical therapy: The vacuum device is the most commonly available mechanical therapy.

- Surgical therapy: Penile prostheses, arterial revascularization, and venous leak surgery have all been employed.

Other therapies, such as **trazodone** and **yohimbine,** are available but are not recommended as first-line therapies for erectile dysfunction. Apomorphine SL is currently available in some markets, but not in the United States. A variety of oral, topical, and injection therapies are currently awaiting FDA approval or are under investigation (see Question 84).

34. My testosterone level is low. Should I receive supplemental testosterone?

At this point in time, the prime **indication** (rationale) for testosterone supplementation is a low testosterone level associated with decreased libido (sexual motivation, thoughts, and feelings). Areas of sexual function that are improved with testosterone therapy include sexual desire, spontaneous sexual thoughts, interest in erotic stimuli, frequency of daytime and nighttime erections, volume of ejaculate and duration, and magnitude and frequency of penile erections during sleep (nocturnal erections).

The effect of testosterone therapy on erectile function is not fully understood. Some evidence suggests that testosterone replacement therapy in men with low testosterone levels improves erectile function either indirectly by improving their libido or directly by improving vascular function in the penis. Studies have demonstrated that men with low normal testosterone levels who fail to respond to oral therapies for erectile dysfunction may ultimately respond to these therapies

Treatment

Vardenafil (Levitra)

An oral form of erectile dysfunction therapy; a phosphodiesterase type 5 inhibitor.

Tadalafil (Cialis)

An oral therapy for erectile dysfunction; a phosphodiesterase type 5 inhibitor with a long half-life (17–21 hours).

Caverject

A form of injection therapy produced by Pharmacia & Upjohn. It contains prostaglandin E_1.

Edex

Alprostadil alfadex. A form of injection therapy produced by Schwarz Pharma. It contains prostaglandin E_1 and works via the same mechanism as Caverject.

Prostaglandin E_1

A type of prostaglandin that increases the cAMP level, which causes smooth-muscle relaxation.

Trazodone

A psychiatric medication that has been reported to cause priapism. Studies using trazodone for the treatment of erectile dysfunction have produced conflicting results. Currently, trazodone is not believed to be a reliable therapy for the treatment of erectile dysfunction.

Yohimbine

An oral medication that acts primarily in the brain. It has been reported to improve erectile function; however, study results are conflicting, and yohimbine is not recommended as a first-line therapy for erectile dysfunction.

Indication

The reason for doing something.

Occult

Not detectable on gross examination.

Digital rectal examination (DRE)

The examination of the prostate by placing a gloved finger into the rectum.

when they are supplemented with testosterone. If your testosterone level is normal, there is no advantage to taking additional testosterone. "Supercharging" you will not necessarily improve your libido.

35. What are the benefits and risks of testosterone therapy?

The main benefit of testosterone therapy is the improvement in serum testosterone level and consequently increased libido. Other theoretical benefits include preservation or improvement in bone mass, which serves to prevent osteoporosis and bone fractures; increased muscle mass and strength, which improves stamina and physical function; decreased cardiovascular disease risk, which improves mood and one's general sense of well-being; and improvement in some aspects of cognition.

Probably the most significant risk associated with testosterone therapy is the chance that it will cause the growth of a clinically **occult** (one that is not detected by gross examination) prostate cancer. Prostate cancer is a hormone-sensitive cancer. Removal of the male hormone, testosterone, has been shown to shrink prostate cancer and slow the growth of prostate cancer. The concern with giving testosterone, even if it is administered only to restore the testosterone level to normal, is the risk of stimulating the growth of an occult prostate cancer. For this reason, men who are considering testosterone therapy should have a **digital rectal examination (DRE)** and a serum PSA both before they start therapy and periodically thereafter.

Testosterone therapy may also stimulate the growth of benign prostate **tissue**. If the amount of this growth is significant, it could lead to changes in voiding function, such as the need to urinate more often, getting up at night more often to urinate, a decrease in the force of the urine stream, or hesitancy with starting the urine stream, to mention but a few of the possible symptoms of an enlarged prostate.

Two notable risks of testosterone therapy are an increase in the number of red blood cells (erythrocytosis) and an increase in the total red cell blood mass (**polycythemia**). These changes are some of the more commonly encountered side effects of testosterone therapy. The risk of their development appears to depend on both the dose of testosterone given and the man's age. **Intramuscular (IM)** testosterone therapy has a higher rate of erythrocytosis than patch or gel (**transdermal**) therapy. Polycythemia and erythrocytosis, if significant, can cause sludging of the blood and worsening of heart disease. If severe, they may require phlebotomy (removal of blood) to counteract their effects. For this reason, periodic checks of your blood count are needed when you are on testosterone therapy.

Other risks of testosterone therapy include an elevation in liver function **enzymes** if testosterone is given orally, breast enlargement, fluid retention, new or worsened sleep apnea, and possibly a higher risk for cardiovascular disease. The effects of testosterone therapy on cardiovascular risk are not fully known, but epidemiologic studies have not shown any increased cardiovascular risk with testosterone therapy. Also, if testosterone is given in large quantities, it may lead to decreased sperm production, causing problems with fertility.

Treatment

Tissue

A specific type of material in the body (e.g., muscle, hair).

Polycythemia

An increase in the total red blood cell mass in the blood.

Intramuscular (IM)

Pertaining to the muscles; injection into the muscle.

Transdermal

Entering through the skin, as in administration of a drug applied to the skin in an ointment, gel, or patch form.

Enzyme

A chemical that is produced by living cells that causes chemical reactions to occur while not being changed itself.

Testosterone therapy is not recommended in certain men and, if used in these populations, should be monitored carefully. These groups include men with a history of prostate cancer or breast cancer, existing polycythemia, sleep apnea, significant symptoms of **benign prostatic hyperplasia** (**BPH**—noncancerous enlargement of the prostate), and **congestive heart failure**.

36. What are the types of testosterone that I can use?

Oral Testosterone Therapy

Currently, oral testosterone therapy is not used in the United States. The oral forms that are available in the United States provide erratic levels of **androgens** (male hormones) and carry a risk of liver toxicity; thus they are not recommended. In other countries, an oral form of testosterone (testosterone undecenoate) is available that is well tolerated and provides more consistent testosterone levels.

Parenteral (Intramuscular) Testosterone Therapy

Parenteral (taken by a route other than the mouth) testosterone has been available for a much longer period than oral testosterone. This form is inexpensive and safe, but has several disadvantages. Use of parenteral testosterone requires periodic deep intramuscular (IM—into the muscle) injections, usually every 2 to 3 weeks. Use of testosterone injection therapy results in **supraphysiologic** (higher than normal) levels of testosterone, usually within 3 days of the shot. These levels steadily decline over the next 10–14 days, with a low

Benign prostatic hyperplasia (BPH)

Noncancerous enlargement of the prostate.

Congestive heart failure

An inability of the heart to pump blood adequately, leading to swelling and fluid in the lungs.

Androgens

Hormones that are necessary for the development and function of the male sexual organs and male sexual characteristics (e.g., hair, voice change).

Parenteral

Administered not by mouth but rather by injection by some other route (e.g., intramuscular, subcutaneous)

Supraphysiologic

Higher than the normal functional state or level in the body.

level occurring around the time of the next injection. This peak-and-trough effect can affect one's mood, well-being, and sexual interest; in some men, these fluctuations can be disturbing. The risk of developing erythrocytosis (increased number of red blood cells) is 44% with injection therapy compared to only 3–18% with transdermal (gel or patch) therapy. Lastly, high peaks in testosterone levels are associated with negative effects on sperm production, so caution is warranted when treating men who are interested in having children with IM testosterone therapy. The recommended dose of intramuscular testosterone is 200–400 mg every 10–21 days to maintain normal average testosterone levels.

Transdermal Testosterone Therapy

Two forms of transdermal testosterone therapy are available: patch and gel.

Transdermal testosterone patch therapy (**Testoderm, Testoderm TTS, and Androderm**) provides one of the most **physiologic** restorations of testosterone level—meaning that the therapy brings your testosterone level back to levels resembling the natural amount of testosterone that should be in your body throughout the day. Transdermal testosterone therapy (therapy that enters through the skin) can be given as a scrotal patch or a nonscrotal patch. The limitations of the scrotal patch (Testoderm) make it less appealing: Its use requires shaving the scrotum—and in some men, the scrotum may be too small to apply the patch. The nonscrotal patch (Androderm, Testoderm TTS) must be applied to a non–hair-bearing skin surface and one to which pressure is not applied (i.e., you cannot put the patch on your buttocks because pressure would be applied

Testoderm

A topical form (patch) of testosterone used for testosterone replacement therapy.

Androderm

A topical form (patch) of testosterone used for testosterone replacement therapy.

Physiologic

Functioning in a normal range for human physiology.

when you sit down). Also, the site of patch placement must be rotated each day.

The testosterone patch is usually applied at bedtime and produces the highest testosterone level in the morning and the lowest level at the time of next patch application; this pattern matches the variation in testosterone levels normally seen over the course of a day. Unlike with the parenteral form of testosterone, the transdermal form has little effect on the blood cell count. The most common side effects of the patch are skin related and may vary from skin irritation to a chemical burn. Application of triamcinolone cream to the skin underneath the patch reservoir decreases the incidence of skin irritation.

The Androderm patch is available in 2.5 mg and 5 mg versions. The usual daily dose is 5 mg, but individual dosing will vary with testosterone levels. The skin patch achieves normal testosterone levels in 67% to 90% of men.

Androgel

A gel form of testosterone replacement therapy.

Testim

A gel form of testosterone replacement therapy.

Another form of transdermal testosterone therapy is a topical gel applied to the skin (**Androgel, Testim**). Gel therapy produces normal testosterone levels in 87% of men. Androgel is available as a 5 g gel packet that delivers 5 mg of testosterone daily. The usual starting dose is 5 g, but the dose may be increased to 7.5 g or 10 g, depending on the individual's original serum testosterone levels. Testim is also a 5 g dose (the gel contains 50 mg of testosterone, but only 10% of it is delivered through the skin); its dose also may be increased to 10 g based on the individual's serum testosterone levels. A testosterone level is usually checked about 2 weeks after starting gel therapy.

Like the patch form of testosterone, the gel is applied once daily. Once applied, it is important to make sure that the gel has completely dried prior to wiping the affected area. You should not shower or swim shortly after the gel is applied. You must also be careful about physical contact when the gel is first applied, because it may be absorbed by your partner if it gets onto your partner's skin. The gel therapy is easy to use and does not cause skin irritation, but it is more expensive than some other forms of testosterone therapy.

Buccal Therapy

Recently, a transbuccal form of testosterone therapy has been approved by the U.S. Food and Drug Administration (FDA), called **Striant.** This buccal system contains 30 mg of testosterone and is used twice each day, in the morning and in the evening. This method of testosterone administration most closely mimics the normal daily variation in testosterone levels. Although Striant is easy to use, it may cause some gum irritation. In one study, 97% of men had a normal testosterone level when taking transbuccal therapy.

Striant

A transbuccal form of testosterone replacement therapy.

37. How should I be monitored while I'm receiving testosterone therapy?

Before starting testosterone therapy, you should undergo a digital rectal examination (DRE—an examination of the prostate in which the physician places a gloved finger into the rectum) and have a prostate-specific antigen (PSA) level taken if you have not had these tests performed recently. If the results of either of these tests are abnormal, then a **transrectal ultrasound**–guided **biopsy**—in which small samples of tissue are removed from the prostate for examination

Transrectal ultrasound

Visualization of the prostate by the use of an ultrasound probe placed into the rectum.

Biopsy

The removal of small sample(s) of tissue for examination under the microscope.

under the microscope—should be performed to rule out prostate cancer before you start testosterone therapy. The presence or suspicion of prostate cancer is a contraindication to testosterone therapy.

A follow-up serum testosterone level should be checked once you begin testosterone therapy to ensure that you are achieving normal levels of testosterone. In addition, your red blood cell count should be checked after 1 month of therapy and periodically thereafter to ensure that the count is not rising. Liver function tests should be performed on a yearly basis. A DRE should be performed and a PSA obtained every 6–12 months to confirm that there are no changes in either's results. If the PSA increases significantly or if the results of the DRE change, the testosterone replacement therapy should be withheld and a transrectal ultrasound-guided prostate biopsy should be performed.

38. How is premature ejaculation treated?

Treatment of premature ejaculation consists of behavioral or medical therapy. Behavioral therapy focuses on "start-stop" or "squeeze" techniques, whereby the man tries to prevent release of the ejaculate. Although such techniques have initial success rates as high as 95%, they tend not to work over the long term. In fact, their success rate is only 25% when assessed 3 years after treatment. Nevertheless, behavioral therapy is important in the initial management of premature ejaculation.

Oral therapy is the most common treatment for premature ejaculation. The medications used are actually antidepressants—either clomipramine (Anafranil) or members of a class of antidepressants called selective serotonin reuptake inhibitor (SSRIs) drugs. Fluoxetine (Prozac) and paroxetine (Paxil) are the two SSRIs that are most commonly used for premature ejaculation; another medication that has also been used for this purpose is sertraline (Zoloft). Clomipramine is the most commonly studied therapy for premature ejaculation. It has been used in doses ranging from 25–50 mg on as-needed, daily, and every-other-day schedules. Side effects of clomipramine include dry mouth, constipation, and feeling "different." With the 50-mg dose, nausea, sleep disturbance, fatigue, and hot flashes are infrequently noted. Sertraline, which is taken in doses ranging from 25–50 mg, is another drug that has been shown to increase the time to ejaculation. Side effects of sertraline are uncommon but may include transient **anorexia** (loss of appetite) and headache. Likewise, fluoxetine and paroxetine, in doses of 20–40 mg per day, have been shown to have beneficial effects on premature ejaculation. The side effects of these medications include nausea, headache, dry mouth, and dizziness.

Anorexia
Loss of appetite.

Topical anesthetic gels such as EMLA can also be used to decrease penile sensitivity. These gels should be placed on the penis and kept in contact with the skin by using a condom over the gel for about 30 minutes. The cream should be washed off before intercourse because it may affect a female partner's vaginal sensitivity.

39. How is retrograde ejaculation treated?

In some individuals, retrograde ejaculation may be treated with medications such as ephedrine (pseudoephedrine, Sudafed, 30–60 mg) or antidepressants, such as desipramine (Norpramine, 50 mg), taken 1 to 2 hours before sexual activity. If the patient has undergone surgery on the bladder outlet, this therapy is less likely to be effective. In men who wish to have children, the sperm can be retrieved from the urine, processed, and used for assisted reproduction.

40. How is anejaculation treated?

Electroejaculation

Use of an electrical stimulus to induce ejaculation.

Anesthesia

The loss of feeling or sensation. With respect to surgery, it means the loss of sensation of pain, as it is induced to allow surgery or other painful procedures to be performed. *General anesthesia* is a state of unconsciousness, produced by anesthetic agents, that is marked by the absence of pain sensation over the entire body and a greater or lesser degree of muscle relaxation. *Local anesthesia* is confined to one part of the body. *Spinal anesthesia* is produced by injection of a local anesthetic into the subarachnoid space around the spinal cord.

In some patients who have suffered spinal cord injury and experience anejaculation, ejaculation may be induced by the application of a vibrator to the penis. In other patients with this condition, **electroejaculation** may be necessary. Electroejaculation often requires **anesthesia** and involves the placement of a probe into the rectum to induce ejaculation. This technique would be used to obtain ejaculate fluid for assisted reproduction; it would not be part of routine sexual activity.

41. How is anorgasmia treated?

Anorgasmia is the inability to experience an orgasm during sex. Congenital anorgasmia is a rare condition that is believed to be related to an overstrict upbringing. In these men, nocturnal emissions ("wet dreams") may occur, but repression of the normal sexual responses prevents the individual from achieving climax and ejaculation. In this situation, psychotherapy may help, as may the use of a vibrator.

Acquired anorgasmia may be caused by medical therapy. Fluoxetine (Prozac), for example, has been associated with delayed ejaculation and an absence of orgasm in as many as 40% of patients who take this medication. Changing to a different antidepressant may lead to an improvement in ejaculatory and orgasmic function. In some individuals with orgasmic dysfunction, changes in their techniques of tactile stimulation may help with the orgasmic dysfunction.

42. How is priapism treated?

Two types of priapism are distinguished: (1) **high-flow priapism,** which is the result of increased blood flow into the penis, and (2) **low-flow priapism,** which is related to decreased penile venous outflow. High-flow priapism does not cause damage to the penis, but low-flow priapism does. More specifically, low-flow priapism may make it more difficult or sometimes impossible to achieve an erection in the future. Therefore, low-flow priapism requires urgent treatment.

The treatment of high-flow priapism focuses on stopping the inflow of blood through the abnormal artery. This can be achieved in one of two ways: by injecting a chemical into the penis that tells the arteries to close down or by **occluding** the abnormal artery. Specialized radiologists, for example, are able to identify the abnormal artery and inject a substance or device into the artery to block it off. Because more than one artery supplies blood to the penis, this **embolization** does not usually cause any damage to the penis or to subsequent erections.

If treated early, low-flow priapism can be treated with the injection of a medication into the side of the penis. If the man waits too long and the rigidity has lasted longer than 6 hours, then a physician must first wash out the stagnant blood from the penis before injecting the chemical that stops the erectile process. In certain

High-flow priapism

Priapism that occurs secondary to increased arterial flow.

Low-flow priapism

Priapism that occurs secondary to venous outflow obstruction.

High-flow priapism does not cause damage to the penis, but low-flow priapism may make it more difficult or sometimes impossible to achieve an erection in the future. Low-flow priapism requires urgent treatment.

Occlusion

Blockage of flow.

Embolization

The introduction of a substance into a blood vessel in an attempt to obstruct (occlude) it.

Treatment

cases, surgical treatment is required to bring the erection down.

43. How is Peyronie's disease treated?

Indications for treatment of Peyronie's disease include penile pain, curvature that prevents penetration, and/or associated erectile dysfunction. Because the exact cause of Peyronie's disease is not known, the best form of therapy for this condition has not been definitively determined. Many therapies are being employed that are based on the theoretical causes of Peyronie's disease and their effects on tissue healing. Medical therapy is most appropriate during the acute (early) phase of Peyronie's disease and includes oral therapy—such as vitamin E, colchicine, tamoxifen, and aminobenzoate potassium (Potaba)—as well as intralesional injections—such as calcium-channel blockers (i.e., verapamil), steroids, and collagenases.

Vitamin E is the traditional initial treatment of choice for Peyronie's disease. This antioxidant can decrease the buildup of harmful chemicals that can injure tissues. Vitamin E is inexpensive, easy to take, and better than placebo for treating pain. (A **placebo** is a fake medication or treatment that has no effect on the body but is often used in experimental studies to determine whether another medication or treatment has an effect.) If the appropriate dose is taken, vitamin E causes no side effects. It has been used in doses ranging from 200 to 800 IU on a daily basis. Because of its ability to increase your risk of bleeding, you should consult your primary care doctor before taking higher doses of this vitamin.

Placebo

A fake medication ("sugar pill") or treatment that has no effect on the body and that is often used in experimental studies to determine whether the experimental medication/treatment has an effect.

Aminobenzoate potassium (Potaba) is another oral therapy that is used primarily for the pain associated with Peyronie's disease. The initial results of a **randomized,** placebo-controlled study using Potaba demonstrated a greater decrease in plaque size with Potaba compared with placebo (32.5% versus 12.5%, respectively) and a larger decrease in penile deviation with Potaba. This drug has a number of drawbacks, however: Unlike vitamin E, it is expensive ($1000 per year), has gastrointestinal side effects, and requires taking 12 g per day. Each tablet includes 0.5 g of medication, so a patient must take four tablets six times daily (a total of 24 tablets), which can be difficult for some patients.

Tamoxifen, which decreases inflammation, has also been used in men with Peyronie's disease. In small studies, an improvement was noted in 55% of men with Peyronie's disease who were treated with tamoxifen at an oral dose of 20 mg for a 3-month period. Tamoxifen tended to work better in men whose Peyronie's disease was not long-standing.

Colchicine, a medication that is used for gout, has been prescribed for Peyronie's disease as well. Small studies have demonstrated a decrease in plaque size in 20% to 50% of men with Peyronie's disease who took it, and a decrease in penile curvature and improvement in the pain in almost 80% of those with pain. Side effects of colchicine include gastrointestinal upset and diarrhea. The doses used range from 0.6 mg to 1.2 mg twice a day for 3 to 5 months.

Other therapies have focused on injecting chemicals into the plaque to promote its breakdown. Such intralesional therapies include collagenase and verapamil (a

Randomized

The process of assigning patients to different forms of treatment in a research study in a random manner.

Treatment

calcium-channel blocker). Studies have shown as much as a 42% improvement in the penile deformity caused by Peyronie's disease with verapamil. Minimal side effects are associated with intralesional injection of verapamil.

Surgical for Peyronie's disease is not a first-line treatment, but rather is usually performed only after the disease stabilizes (i.e., the disease has been present for a year or longer). The surgical treatment of Peyronie's disease consists of either correction of the penile curvature or placement of a penile prosthesis to straighten the penis and allow for erections in men who have penile curvature and erectile dysfunction.

Surgical treatment of the penile curvature of Peyronie's disease may be performed in two ways:

- *Removal (excision) of the plaque and replacement of that segment of tunica with another piece of tissue—that is, a graft.* The advantage of this technique is that it maintains penile length. Potential disadvantages of the plaque excision and grafting technique include residual curvature or contracture, shrinkage of the graft requiring another procedure, and postoperative onset of erectile dysfunction. The occurrence of erectile dysfunction after the plaque excision and grafting may be related to damage to the underlying penile tissue during the surgery, lack of compliance of the graft, or development of a venous leak.

- *Taking a tuck of the tunica on the side of the penis opposite the plaque.* This technique leads to shortening of the penis; the extent of the shortening depends on the size of the tuck, called a Nesbit plication. In most cases, the small amount of shortening is not noticeable and does not affect sexual function or the ability to stand to void.

When significant penile curvature and erectile dysfunction are present, a penile prosthesis (see Question 65) is an option that can treat both problems. At the time the prosthesis is placed, the penis is straightened by the "modeling technique." This technique involves bending of the erect penis in the direction opposite to the curvature (the prosthesis is inflated at the time). The prosthesis is inflated before the procedure is completed to ensure that the penis has been satisfactorily straightened. On rare occasions, another procedure, such as corporal grafting, is needed in addition to placement of the prosthesis to achieve adequate straightening. The patient can also perform some modeling after the prosthesis has been placed to straighten the penis even more. Again, this would be done with the penis erect and would involve bending it in the direction opposite to the curvature. The technique, risks, and satisfaction rate associated with prosthesis placement are discussed in the section on penile prostheses.

44. What are oral therapies for erectile dysfunction—specifically, the phosphodiesterase type 5 (PDE-5) inhibitors?

Currently, three oral therapies are available for the treatment of erectile dysfunction. The first therapy to become available was sildenafil (Pfizer's Viagra), which was approved by the FDA in 1998. Vardenafil (Bayer's Levitra) and tadalafil (Lily Icos's Cialis) were approved for use years later. All three of these oral therapies are **phosphodiesterase type 5 (PDE-5) inhibitors.**

Phosphodiesterase type 5 (PDE-5) inhibitor

A chemical that prevents the function of PDE-5. The use of such an inhibitor leads to an increase in cGMP.

To understand how these therapies work, it is important to review the process involved in the normal erection. When aroused or stimulated sexually, the brain sends out messages (neurotransmitters), which result in the release of a chemical—nitric oxide—from nerves in the pelvis (see Question 4). The nitric oxide then stimulates the production of the chemical called cGMP, which in turn tells the cavernosal muscle in the penis to relax, thereby allowing more blood to flow into the penis. cGMP is broken down in the penis by an enzyme, **phosphodiesterase type 5 (PDE-5).** Thus, if PDE-5 is prevented from working by administration of a PDE-5 inhibitor, there will be more cGMP present and thus a greater stimulus for increased blood flow.

Phosphodiesterase type 5 (PDE-5)

An enzyme that is responsible for the breakdown of cGMP. Inhibition of PDE-5 leads to a buildup of cGMP.

Critical to the success of all of the PDE-5 inhibitors is the need for sexual arousal (sexual stimulation) after taking the medication. That is, these medications will not cause an erection to occur without sexual stimulation. It is okay to have a glass of wine, a beer, or a mixed drink when using these therapies—such limited alcohol consumption should not interfere with their effectiveness. Too much alcohol, however, may have a negative effect on erectile function, so a man should limit his alcohol intake when taking any of these medications.

Critical to the success of all of the PDE-5 inhibitors is the need for sexual arousal (sexual stimulation) after taking the medication.

45. Who is a candidate for oral therapy with a PDE-5 inhibitor?

Most men can take PDE-5 inhibitors. Nevertheless, there are certain contraindications to the use of these therapies. If these limitations are ignored, serious or even life-threatening problems may occur.

Specific contraindications to the use of PDE-5 inhibitors include the use of products containing organic **nitrates,** such as sublingual **nitroglycerin,** amyl nitrates, nitroglycerin patches, and long-acting nitrates such as Imdur (Table 3). Nitrates (e.g., nitroglycerin), which are a form of nitric acid that causes opening of the blood vessels to the heart, and nitrites should not be used for angina for at least 24 hours after a man has taken a PDE-5 inhibitor: When combined, nitrates and PDE-5 inhibitors may significantly lower blood pressure to a potentially life-threatening level. For this reason, a contradiction to the use of PDE-5 inhibitors is unstable angina requiring frequent use of short-acting or sublingual nitroglycerin.

Should you experience chest pain during intercourse, you should stop what you are doing. If the pain persists, you should go to the emergency room and notify the personnel there that you took a PDE-5 inhibitor so that they will know not to give you any form of nitrate.

The use of PDE-5 inhibitors has not been studied in patients with the following conditions, so caution should be used in treating such individuals with a PDE-5 inhibitor:

- Congestive heart failure (the inability of the heart to pump blood adequately, which leads to swelling and fluid in the lungs) with a borderline low blood volume.

- Recent heart attack (myocardial infarction).

- **Hypotension**

Nitrate

A form of nitric acid that causes dilation (opening up) of the blood vessels to the heart. Nitroglycerin is a form of nitrate.

Nitroglycerin

A medication that is usually taken sublingually (under the tongue) for the relief of angina. It may also be applied to the chest in a paste form for the prevention of angina.

Hypotension

Low blood pressure.

Treatment

- Tadalafil (Cialis): If using an alpha blocker, the individual must be on stable alpha-blocker therapy first and then start with the lowest dose of tadalafil.

46. How do I use PDE-5 inhibitors?

Use of PDE-5 inhibitors is "on demand," meaning that in most cases, each time you want to have intercourse, you need to take a pill. These pills facilitate your body's response, rather than causing an erection on their own, so they require sexual stimulation or foreplay to work. Other medications that increase PDE-5 inhibitor levels include erythromycin (E-mycin), clarithromycin (Biaxin), ketoconazole (Nizoral), itraconazole (Sporanox), and cimetidine (Tagamet). Men taking protease inhibitors, such as indinavir (Crixivan), nelfinavir (Viracept), ritonavir (Norvir), or saquinavir (Fortovase), should start at a lower dose and take the PDE-5 inhibitor less frequently because the protease inhibitors (generally prescribed for HIV infection and AIDS) increase the blood levels of the PDE-5 inhibitors.

The three PDE-5 inhibitors vary somewhat in terms of how far in advance a man needs to take the medication for it to be effective and how long after taking the medication he can anticipate a response. Both sildenafil (Viagra) and vardenafil (Levitra) should be taken about 1 hour prior to intercourse, whereas tadalafil (Cialis) should be taken 2 hours prior to anticipated intercourse. Diet may affect the results with sildenafil—specifically, an individual should avoid consuming a high-fat meal prior to using this drug. Tadalafil has a long half-life (17–21 hours); thus, if this medication works for you, it may work for as long as 3 days after you initially take the medication. This is not the case for all men.

Multiple doses are available for each of these medications, but it is recommended that you start at the lowest dose and titrate the dose upward as needed. In certain patients, a lower dose and less frequent use of the medication are recommended. Your doctor will tell you which dose and dosing interval is appropriate for you. All of the PDE-5 inhibitors should be taken only once in a 24-hour period.

All of the PDE-5 inhibitors should be taken only once in a 24-hour period.

47. What is the success rate for PDE-5 inhibitors?

Overall, the PDE-5 inhibitors have a similar success rate. Individuals who have failed to respond to one of these medications may, however, respond to a different PDE-5 inhibitor. Similarly, if you experience bothersome side effects with one PDE-5 inhibitor, it is worthwhile trying another option.

Sildenafil (Viagra) has been approved for use for the longest period of time, and thus the most data are available regarding the use of this PDE-5 inhibitor. The success rate for sildenafil ranges from 48% to 81% and varies with the cause of the erectile dysfunction (Table 4).

Vardenafil (Levitra) has been shown to be an effective oral therapy for use in erectile dysfunction. With this medication, improvements in ability to penetrate have been noted in 75–80% of men and ability to maintain an erection in 64–65%. In one study, vardenafil was shown to be helpful in patients who had previously failed to respond to sildenafil therapy.

Table 4   Success of Viagra by Cause of Erectile Dysfunction

Etiology	Success rate	Source(s) and studies
General population	70%	N Engl J Med 1998;338:1397–1404 Urology 1999;S3:800–805
Hypertension	70%	N Engl J Med 1998;338:1397–1404
Spinal cord injury	57–93%	Eur Urol 2000;38:134–193 Neurology 1998;51:1629–1633
Spina bifida (myelomeningocele)	80%	J Urol 2000;164(3, part 2):958–961
Multiple sclerosis	90%	Urol Clin N Am 2001;32:289–308
Psychogenic: depression and antidepressent treat- ment related	73–89%	Int J Impot Res 1998;10:53, 254a
Bilateral nerve-sparing radical prostatectomy	32–80%	Int J Impot Res 2001;13(Suppl 5):568
Radiation for prostate cancer	70–80%	Urology 2001;57:769–773 J Clin Oncol 1999;17:3444–3449
Diabetes mellitus	50–65%	JAMA 1999;281:421–426

Tadalafil (Cialis) has been shown to have a 62–77% success rate in terms of ability to penetrate and a 50–64% success rate in terms of ability to maintain an erection. In a group of 1100 men from five controlled studies, a 61% erection success rate was noted with the 10-mg tablets, and a 73% erection success rate was noted with the 20-mg tablets. Unlike the other PDE-5 inhibitors, tadalafil has a long half-life and thus may continue to be effective for as long as 3 days in some individuals.

Spinal Cord Injury and Spina Bifida

Patients whose erectile dysfunction is caused by spinal cord injury or spina bifida (a congenital condition affecting the spinal cord, also called myelomeningocele) frequently respond to 25–50 mg of sildenafil. Men with complete spinal cord injuries tend to require higher doses than those with incomplete lesions. Vardenafil has also been shown to be effective in men with erectile dysfunction secondary to spinal cord injury. In one study, 76% of the men were able to penetrate their partner and 59% were able to maintain an erection when they took this drug. Tadalafil has also been demonstrated to be effective in patients with spinal cord injury.

Diabetes Mellitus

The effectiveness of sildenafil in men with diabetes mellitus–related erectile dysfunction does not appear to be affected by the patient's age, duration of the erectile dysfunction, or duration of the diabetes mellitus. In addition, the **glycosylated hemoglobin** (hemoglobin A_{1c}, a chemical in the blood that allows blood sugar control to be monitored) levels and the prevalence of peripheral neuropathy do not affect patients' response to Viagra. In patients with type 1 and 2 diabetes, a preliminary study showed that 85% of the men using the 10- and 20-mg doses of vardenafil noted an improvement in erectile function, compared to 13% of the men taking placebo.

Glycosylated hemoglobin

A chemical in the blood that allows monitoring of blood sugar control in individuals with diabetes mellitus. An elevated $HgbA_{1c}$ is indicative of poor blood sugar control.

Dialysis

Studies have shown that sildenafil can restore erectile function in 60% of men with erectile dysfunction who are on hemodialysis and continuous ambulatory peritoneal dialysis. In this group, the drug was also well tolerated.

Penile Prosthesis

Sildenafil has been shown to increase sexual satisfaction in men with inflatable penile prostheses. By inducing dilation and engorgement of the residual corporeal erectile tissue as well as the glans (tip) of the penis, this medication can complement the erection obtained from the penile prosthesis.

External-Beam Radiation Therapy

The response rate for sildenafil in men who have undergone external-beam radiation therapy (EBRT) exceeds 70%. Men who note some—albeit inadequate—erectile function after EBRT have response rates as high as 90% with sildenafil, whereas those who do not note any erections at all after EBRT have a 52% response rate with this PDE-5 inhibitor. Most men require the 100-mg dose.

Tadalafil has also been shown to be effective in men with EBRT-related erectile dysfunction. In one study, 67% reported improved erections and 48% reported successful intercourse after taking this medication.

After Radical Prostatectomy

Satisfaction rates with sildenafil (Viagra) used as therapy for post–radical prostatectomy erectile dysfunction range from 15–80%. Preoperative erectile function, the nerve-sparing nature of the surgery, and the timing of sildenafil administration are all factors that affect response rates. As would be expected, the best success rates occur in men who experienced adequate erectile function before surgery and who underwent a **bilateral** nerve-sparing radical prostatectomy. The worst success rates are observed in men who had erectile dysfunction before surgery and in those who had a non–nerve-

Bilateral

Affecting both sides.

sparing **radical prostatectomy.** The success rates of sildenafil for men who have undergone a bilateral nerve-sparing radical prostatectomy are approximately 70%; for those who have undergone a unilateral nerve-sparing radical prostatectomy, they are approximately 50%; and for those who have undergone a non–nerve-sparing radical prostatectomy, the success rates are approximately 15%.

Studies have shown that erectile dysfunction may improve in men after radical prostatectomy during the first year or two following their surgery. Lack of erections, both sexually aroused and nocturnal, after radical prostatectomy has been associated with penile fibrosis and loss of penile length over the long term.

Exciting studies evaluating the benefit of consistent use of sildenafil or injection therapy to promote penile blood flow after radical prostatectomy are being evaluated. It is hoped that enhancing tissue oxygenation will minimize scarring and perhaps lead to earlier recovery of erectile function or improved response to therapy.

In a study that surveyed men using a **global assessment questionnaire (GAQ),** 59.4% of men taking 10 mg of vardenafil and 65.2% of men taking 20 mg of vardenafil reported having a favorable response to the medication. For the men who had undergone bilateral nerve-sparing radical prostatectomy, 70% of those taking 20 mg of vardenafil reported having a favorable response. In men with erectile dysfunction after a bilateral nerve-sparing radical prostatectomy, 20 mg of tadalafil was associated with a 74% improvement in erectile dysfunction, and 52% of men reported having successful intercourse.

Radical prostatectomy

A surgical procedure for prostate cancer in which the entire prostate and seminal vesicles, and part of the vas deferens, are removed.

Erectile dysfunction may improve in men after radical prostatectomy during the first year or two following their surgery.

Global assessment questionnaire (GAQ)

A self-administered questionnaire that allows patients to rate improvement in erectile function.

Other Patient Populations

Sildenafil (Viagra) has been shown to be quite effective in reversing antidepressant-induced sexual dysfunction and antipsychotic-induced sexual dysfunction.

If you have tried a PDE-5 inhibitor but it did not work for you, it is important that you reevaluate how you used the medication. Remember that eating a high-fat diet can affect the delay in the time until the drug becomes effective and lower the absorption of sildenafil. Also, if you tried only a few pills, you may not have given the medication a sufficient trial. Studies have shown that it may take as many as eight trials with the medication (including the need to increase the dose if several attempts at a lower dose are not effective and are not producing significant side effects) before you get a good response. In a similar manner, if you are anxious, concerned, worried, or stressed when you are trying the medication, the PDE-5 inhibitor will not be as effective. It is important for both you and your partner to be as relaxed as possible and to minimize the pressure and anxiety related to concern about whether it will work so that the medication has the best chance of working. Some people advocate taking the pill and participating only in foreplay on several occasions, just to get both you and your partner to relax, and then giving it a complete trial.

48. What are the side effects of PDE-5 inhibitors?

Several side effects are associated with all three of the currently available PDE-5 inhibitors—namely, headache, flushing, nasal congestion, and dyspepsia. Headache, flushing, and nasal congestion are vasodilatory effects and reflect dilation (increased opening) of blood vessels in the head, face, skin of the chest, and nasal mucosa, respectively. Dyspepsia (indigestion) may occur as a result of relaxation of the gastroesophageal sphincter. The gastroesophageal sphincter lies at the junction between the stomach and the esophagus (the tube through which food passes to enter into the stomach after you swallow). With relaxation of the sphincter, reflux (backflow) of acidic stomach contents into the esophagus may occur, causing a sour taste.

Table 5 presents the side effects most commonly encountered with sildenafil (Viagra). With the exception of abnormal vision, these side effects are also noted with tadalafil (Cialis) and vardenafil (Levitra), though their frequency may vary slightly between the different medications. The abnormal vision that can occur with sildenafil use typically involves a change in color vision (abnormal blue/green discrimination) related to the inhibitory effect of sildenafil on phosphodiesterase type 6 in the eye. Other visual disturbances that have been reported include double vision, temporary visual loss, ocular redness, and burning. These side effects are transient, no long-standing changes in the eye or in vision have been reported, and ophthalmologic evaluation of the effects of sildenafil on the eye has not demonstrated any long-term adverse effects. Sildenafil also does not increase intraocular pressure. Similar visual disturbances are not reported in patients taking tadalafil or vardenafil (Levitra). Myalgia has been reported in 1–3% of men taking tadalafil, however, though this effect is usually responsive to nonsteroidal anti-inflammatory medications such as ibuprofen.

All three of the currently marketed PDE-5 inhibitors may cause mild, transient decreases in blood pressure. In

All three of the currently marketed PDE-5 inhibitors (sildenafil, vardenafil, and tadalafil) may cause mild, transient decreases in blood pressure.

Table 5   Side Effects Associated with Viagra

	No. of Patients Reporting an Adverse Event (%)	
	Viagra (n = 734)	Placebo (n = 725)
Headache	15.3	3.9
Flushing	10.5	0.7
Dyspepsia	6.5	1.7
Nasal congestion	4.2	1.5
Respiratory tract infection	4.2	5.4
Flu syndrome	33	2.9
Urinary tract infection	3.1	1.5
Altered vision	2.7	0.4
Diarrhea	2.6	1.0
Dizziness	2.2	1.2
Rash	2.2	1.4
Back pain	2.2	1.7
Arthralgia	2.0	1.5

Reprinted with permission from Carson C, Kirby R, Goldstein I. Textbook of Erectile Dysfunction. Oxford, UK: Isis Medical Media, 1999, Table 26.4, p. 304.

most cases, such elevations do not cause any side effects. In men who take multiple medications for high blood pressure or those with low blood pressure (hypotension), however, even this mild change in blood pressure may be significant. Similarly, men who take alpha blockers for benign prostate enlargement (BPH—noncancerous enlargement of the prostate) are cautioned about taking PDE-5 inhibitors (see Question 45).

Since the FDA's approval of sildenafil, tadalafil, and vardenafil, a few rare side effects have been reported with these medications. Although none of these side effects is necessarily caused by the PDE-5 inhibitor, patients and doctors should still be aware of them:

- Heart attacks and death. In some cases, these cardiac events are clearly related to the combined use of nitroglycerin-containing products and a PDE-5 inhibitor. Some such events have occurred in men with known cardiovascular disease, but other patients who experienced these problems have not had previously identified cardiovascular disease. Given this fact, men with cardiovascular disease should discuss the risks of PDE-5 inhibitor use with their primary care provider or cardiologist (if they have one) prior to taking the PDE-5 inhibitor. If you are unsure about the status of your cardiovascular health, you should discuss the possibility of further evaluation, such as a stress test, with your primary care provider.

- Stroke.

- Onset of irregular fast heartbeat (atrial fibrillation).

- Priapism. This side effect has been reported on rare occasions with use of PDE-5 inhibitors. If you experience an erection lasting 2 to 3 hours, it is important that you seek immediate care. Failure to obtain treatment in a timely fashion could potentially cause further penile damage.

- **Nonarteritic ischemic optic neuropathy (NAION)** has been reported with all three PDE-5 inhibitors since they entered the market and were used in

Nonarteritic ischemic optic neuropathy (NAION)

A sudden, painless loss of vision in one or both eyes. The cause is reduced blood flow to the optic nerve.

larger groups of patients than had participated in the clinical trials of these drugs. NAION is a sudden, painless loss of vision, which may affect one or both eyes. At this time a cause-and-effect relationship between PDE-5 inhibitor use and NAION has not been established. Several medical conditions that cause erectile dysfunction are also risk factors for NAION, including hypertension, diabetes mellitus, atherosclerosis, and elevated cholesterol. Another condition, crowded disc, also increases the risk of NAION. If you experience a sudden loss of vision when taking a PDE-5 inhibitor, it is recommended that you seek medical attention immediately. A large study that evaluated 52,000 patient-years of observations revealed that the incidence of NAION in men taking sildenafil was similar to that reported in the general population.

Tachyphylaxis

Decreased response of a patient to a drug that was previously effective.

In addition, there have been reports of tachyphylaxis following sildenafil use. **Tachyphylaxis** is the decreased response to a drug after a few doses, such that the medication initially works, but the same dose loses its effectiveness after only a short period of time. It is unclear whether the reported phenomena were truly cases of tachyphylaxis, as opposed to progression of the erectile dysfunction or the effects of dietary indiscretions and improper use of the medication.

49. How do PDE-5 inhibitors compare to other therapies for erectile dysfunction?

Because sildenafil (Viagra) was the first PDE-5 inhibitor approved for use in erectile dysfunction, most of the comparative data available focus on this drug.

Vacuum Device

In a study comparing sildenafil with the vacuum device (see Question 63), two thirds of men who were using the vacuum device successfully and then tried sildenafil elected to continue using the oral medication and stop using the vacuum device.

Intracavernous Injection Therapy

In a study comparing sildenafil with injection therapy (see Question 58), of the men who achieved satisfactory erections with both sildenafil and injection therapy, 73% preferred to use the oral medication. In a study of men who had satisfactory erections using less than 20 µg of **alprostadil** injection therapy (Caverject or Edex), 69% of them successfully changed from injection therapy to sildenafil and decided to continue with this oral medication. Although the success rate with injection therapy was higher in this study, the satisfaction rate was higher for sildenafil.

In another study that examined the use of triple P injection therapy, the dose of triple P needed to obtain an erection correlated with the likelihood of response to sildenafil. If the dose of triple P was between 0.35 cc and 0.6 cc, the success rate with sildenafil was 55%; however, if the dose of triple P required was 0.7 cc, then the success rate with sildenafil was only 20%. Other studies have demonstrated that the patient's response to prior treatments for erectile dysfunction is not a predictor of response to sildenafil.

50. What is intraurethral alprostadil (MUSE)?

Intraurethral alprostadil (Vivus's **MUSE**) is an **intraurethral** medication (i.e., a drug that is injected into the

Alprostadil

Prostaglandin E_1. For the treatment of erectile dysfunction, alprostadil comes in several forms—specifically, a suppository that is placed into the urethra (MUSE) or a liquid form that is delivered by intracavernous injection (Caverject or Edex).

Intraurethral alprostadil

See *MUSE*.

MUSE

Intraurethral alprostadil; a small suppository that comes preloaded in a small applicator that is placed into the tip of the penis. The small button at the other end of the suppository is squeezed to release the suppository into the urethra. Gentle rubbing of the penis causes the suppository to dissolve. The prostaglandin is then absorbed through the urethral mucosa and passes into the corpora cavernosa, where it stimulates blood flow into the penis through the cAMP pathway.

Intraurethral

Placed into the urethra.

urethra) that was approved by the FDA in June 1998. Alprostadil is a synthetic form of a normal body chemical, prostaglandin E_1, that causes increased blood flow into the penis. MUSE works differently than sildenafil (Viagra), the oral therapy for erectile dysfunction. That is, the prostaglandin in MUSE stimulates the production of a chemical called cAMP, which, like cGMP, can cause the relaxation of smooth muscle and thus increase blood flow to the penis.

51. Who is a candidate for MUSE?

There are relatively few contraindications to the use of MUSE. Because MUSE is administered intraurethrally and not all of the dose may be absorbed at the time of ejaculation, you should not use this therapy if your partner is pregnant.

Men who have undergone prior radical prostatectomy appear to have an increased risk of penile or urethral burning with MUSE, and they should be warned about this possibility. The exact cause of this side effect is not known, but it may be caused by a postsurgical supersensitivity of the corpora or increased retention of the MUSE in the penis because the dorsal vein may have been tied off at the time of radical prostatectomy. In particular, patients who have experienced pain with alprostadil in the past are likely to experience discomfort with MUSE. Hypotension (low blood pressure) and **syncope** (fainting) have been noted with MUSE as well and can be associated with serious cardiovascular consequences; for this reason, MUSE should be used with caution in men who have significant cardiovascular risks and in older men. Men who are at increased risk for priapism, such as those with sickle

Syncope

A temporary loss of consciousness.

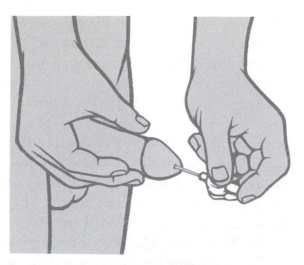

Figure 7   Muse insertion. © 2002 The StayWell Company. Reprinted with permission.

cell anemia, leukemia, polycythemia, thrombo-cythemia, or multiple myeloma, should not use MUSE. Men in whom sexual activity is not advisable, such as those with severe cardiovascular disease, should not use MUSE.

52. How do I use MUSE?

MUSE is an on-demand medication, meaning that you must take it each time that you wish to achieve an erection. The suppository of the alprostadil is enclosed in a small applicator (Figure 7). You should void before inserting the tip of the applicator into your penis, because voiding helps lubricate the urethra. Other top-ical lubricants, such as K-Y Jelly, Vaseline, and mineral oil, cannot be used with MUSE because they interfere with the absorption of the alprostadil. Once the appli-cator is placed into the urethra, you squeeze the small round button at the end, which releases the supposi-tory into the urethra. Gently rocking the applicator from side to side will ensure that the suppository disengages from the applicator and remains within the urethra when the applicator is removed. Once the applicator is removed, gentle massaging of the penis causes the suppository to dissolve in the urethra.

Once in the body, the alprostadil is absorbed through the urethral tissue and travels via blood vessels into the corpora cavernosa (the erectile tissue of the penis). There, it stimulates dilation of the arteries and provides for relaxation of the cavernosal smooth muscle within 10 to 20 minutes. The onset of a response to the MUSE is quick, usually occurring within 7 to 20 minutes after it is administered. The duration of the response varies with the dose and ranges from 60 to 80 minutes.

Several doses of MUSE are available: 125, 250, 500, and 1000 µg. This medication must be refrigerated.

The onset of a response to the MUSE is quick, usually occurring within 7 to 20 minutes after it is administered.

53. What is the success rate of MUSE?

In the initial studies of MUSE's effectiveness, the success rate was 64%. More recent studies have demonstrated its efficacy to be only 30%, however. Attempts to increase this success rate via the use of the ACTIS venous constrictor, a constricting band that is placed the base of the penis, have helped some men. In men, an erection rigid enough for penetration occur in the standing position, however, when individuals change to a supine position, th may decrease. In these men, changing used for intercourse or using the constric proved helpful.

Efficacy

The power or ability to produce an effect.

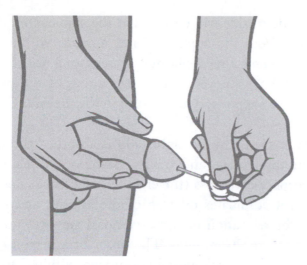

Figure 7   Muse insertion. © 2002 The StayWell Company. Reprinted with permission.

cell anemia, leukemia, polycythemia, thrombo-cythemia, or multiple myeloma, should not use MUSE. Men in whom sexual activity is not advisable, such as those with severe cardiovascular disease, should not use MUSE.

52. How do I use MUSE?

MUSE is an on-demand medication, meaning that you must take it each time that you wish to achieve an erection. The suppository of the alprostadil is enclosed in a small applicator (Figure 7). You should void before inserting the tip of the applicator into your penis, because voiding helps lubricate the urethra. Other topical lubricants, such as K-Y Jelly, Vaseline, and mineral oil, cannot be used with MUSE because they interfere with the absorption of the alprostadil. Once the applicator is placed into the urethra, you squeeze the small round button at the end, which releases the suppository into the urethra. Gently rocking the applicator from side to side will ensure that the suppository disengages from the applicator and remains within the urethra when the applicator is removed. Once the applicator is removed, gentle massaging of the penis causes the suppository to dissolve in the urethra.

Once in the body, the alprostadil is absorbed through the urethral tissue and travels via blood vessels into the corpora cavernosa (the erectile tissue of the penis). There, it stimulates dilation of the arteries and provides for relaxation of the cavernosal smooth muscle within 10 to 20 minutes. The onset of a response to the MUSE is quick, usually occurring within 7 to 20 minutes after it is administered. The duration of the response varies with the dose and ranges from 60 to 80 minutes.

Several doses of MUSE are available: 125, 250, 500, and 1000 µg. This medication must be refrigerated.

The onset of a response to the MUSE is quick, usually occurring within 7 to 20 minutes after it is administered.

53. What is the success rate of MUSE?

In the initial studies of MUSE's effectiveness, the success rate was 64%. More recent studies have demonstrated its **efficacy** to be only 30%, however. Attempts to increase this success rate via the use of the ACTIS venous constrictor, a constricting band that is placed at the base of the penis, have helped some men. In some men, an erection rigid enough for penetration may occur in the standing position; however, when these individuals change to a supine position, the erection may decrease. In these men, changing the position used for intercourse or using the constricting band has proved helpful.

Efficacy

The power or ability to produce an effect.

It is difficult to predict who will and who will not respond to MUSE. The patient's age and the cause of the erectile dysfunction, for example, are not predictive of response. Nevertheless, MUSE is unlikely to be effective in men who have not responded to **intracavernous** injection therapy.

Intracavernous

Into the corpora cavernosa.

54. What are the side effects of MUSE?

The most common side effect, occurring in one third to one half of all men who take MUSE, is pain. This pain may be present in the penis, urethra, testis, or perineum. The intensity of the pain varies according to the dose taken: Thus, as the dose increases, the intensity of the pain may likewise increase. Hypotension and syncopal episodes (temporary loss of consciousness caused by decreased blood flow to the brain) have been reported in 1.2% to 4% of men who took MUSE, with their frequency depending on the dose used. Other side effects include urethral bleeding (in 4% to 5% of men who took MUSE), dizziness (in 1%), and urinary tract infection (in 0.2%). Prolonged erections and penile fibrosis (scarring) rarely occur. Ten percent of female partners experience vaginal irritation or vaginitis.

55. What is penile injection therapy?

Intracavernous injection therapy is the process whereby a small amount of a chemical is injected directly into the corpora cavernosa. These chemicals relax smooth muscle, thereby helping to increase blood flow into the penis. The major advantage of injection therapy is that it does not depend on oral absorption, as pills do, or on absorption through the tissues, as MUSE does. The disadvantage is that it requires a small penile injection. Most men are anxious when they initially start with injection therapy but find that the procedure itself is not especially uncomfortable. In most patients who do not respond to first-line oral therapy or who are not candidates for oral therapy, injection therapy provides satisfactory erections.

The only FDA-approved chemicals for intracavernous injection therapy are Caverject (Pharmacia & Upjohn) and Edex (Schwarz Pharma). Both of these agents consist of prostaglandin E_1. Other agents used alone or in combination include papaverine and phentolamine. All three medications—prostaglandin E_1, papaverine, and phentolamine—may be used in combination, in which case the combination is referred to as "triple P" or "trimix." Prostaglandin E_1 and triple P are the two most common forms of injection therapy used, and each offers a unique set of advantages and disadvantages (see Question 59).

Bob's comment:

Some people resolve their erectile dysfunction through the use of injection therapy—I was, but am no longer, a member of that group. Because I am an insulin-dependent diabetic, I have had much experience with needles. Twice daily, I use an insulin-laden syringe to satiate my body's need to control my sugar levels. There is one big difference between injection therapy for erectile dysfunction and insulin injections for diabetes: With diabetes I inject my arms, legs, or abdomen; with the injection therapy for erectile dysfunction, I inject my penis. To me, that was a big difference.

I was first introduced to injection therapy as a quick means to achieve an erection. The physician primed what seemed to me to be a rather large syringe with the fluid, that, when injected, would cause an erection. I was instructed that this was accomplished by injecting the needle into the side of my penis. Within minutes, voilà, an erection!

Needless to say, I was not overly excited when the instruction and test-dosing were performed in the office, and I was less enthralled when I self-injected at home. In fact, after the first success in the physician's office, subsequent injections at home produced erections that were less firm and ineffective. Upon discussion with my physician, the dosage was increased. However, as we continued to go up and up on the medication, it just didn't seem to improve things. Maybe the problem was related to my diabetes or maybe it was my mind—hard to say. Perhaps the injection itself was my undoing. Preparing for a sexual interlude, I would isolate myself in the bathroom, prepare the syringe, and then administer the injection. How romantic! Many an evening when the atmosphere was ripe for sex, I discreetly (at least I thought I was being discreet) avoided the encounter. Envisioning the syringe and the prep was too much for me. No sale: I preferred to watch the Red Sox.

56. Who is a candidate for penile injection therapy?

Because the injection requires manual dexterity, it is important that the man be able to perform self-injection. In some men for whom giving an injection may be difficult or who are anxious about pushing the needle into the side of their penis, an auto-injector is available that makes this task easier. Another option is to have the man's partner perform the injection. Similarly, if the man is obese and has trouble seeing his penis, self-injection may be difficult, so he would need to enlist the aid of his partner.

If a man has tried MUSE in the past and has experienced significant discomfort with it, then using Caverject or Edex will merely cause further discomfort. In this situation, it would be more appropriate to try triple P. In addition, if the man has a known hypersensitivity or has had a prior reaction to prostaglandins, then Caverject or Edex would not be appropriate. Depending on the severity of the reaction, however, the man might consider using bimix (papaverine and phentolamine only).

In a number of conditions, injection therapy may potentially produce additional side effects. For example, men who are prone to priapism, such as those with sickle cell disease or trait, multiple myeloma, and leukemia, are at increased risk for priapism if they use injection therapy. Men with Peyronie's disease should be aware that the process of injection causes local trauma to the tunica albuginea, which could theoretically cause new plaques to form. Men who are taking blood thinners, such as warfarin (Coumadin), can use injection therapy, but should apply pressure to the injection site for a minute or so to prevent a bruise. Men who are taking a monoamine oxidase inhibitor (an older type of antidepressant), such as Marplan, Nardil, Phenelzine, or Parnate, should not use this therapy.

57. How do I perform penile injection therapy?

Before you start to use intracavernous injection therapy at home, you will receive a test dose in the physician's office. Of all of the therapies available, intracavernous injection therapy carries the highest risk of priapism, with as many as 2% of patients experiencing this side effect. Most cases of priapism occur with first use, during the test dosing. This fact is important because if you return to your urologist's office within 3–4 hours, the erection can easily be brought back down with an injection of another chemical. If your urologist is concerned about priapism, he or she may choose to terminate your erection by injecting you with a chemical to stop the erection before you head home. Thus test dosing minimizes your risk of having a case of priapism at an inopportune time.

Of all of the therapies available, intracavernous injection therapy carries the highest risk of priapism. Test dosing in the physician's office can minimize your risk of having a case of priapism at an inopportune time.

Your urologist can also use the test dosing session as a time for hands-on instruction. That is, you can learn how to inject yourself and actually perform your first self-injection with the physician's guidance in the office. This consideration is very important because the first time you perform the injection therapy at home, you will probably be nervous. Remembering that you performed the injection in the office may help you relax.

The needle that you use to inject the medication is quite short and small. It is short because it does not need to pierce deeply into the penis, just into the corpora on one side, for the therapy to be effective (Figure 8). It is small because you will be injecting only 1 cc or less of medication. After your initial test dose, your urologist will decide on a dose that you will try initially at home. Do not get discouraged if this initial dose is not adequate. Most physicians would prefer to prescribe a dose that is too small and then increase it as needed to avoid priapism.

Treatment

Hold your penis firmly against the side of your thigh.

When doing this, grasp the head of your penis with your thumb and index finger.

Stretch it tautly so it does not skip during the injection.

In uncircumcised men, the foreskin must be pulled back to assure proper placement of the injection.

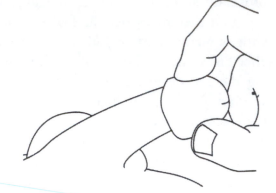

Hold the barrel of the syringe between the thumb and index finger.

To avoid injecting the solution too early, do not put your thumb on the plunger during this step.

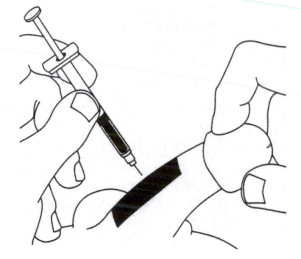

Figure 8   Injection therapy: proper location of injection. Reprinted with permission from Pfizer, Inc.

When using injection therapy at home, you should keep several points in mind:

• Look where you are going to inject the syringe to make sure that no superficial veins are in the area.

• Gently wipe the area with an alcohol swab.

- Always inject the medication on the side of the penis toward the base. The needle should be inserted straight into the penis at a 90-degree angle to the penis.

- Apply pressure to the injection site for a minute or two. If you see any bleeding from the injection site, maintain the pressure for about 5 minutes. Men taking blood thinners should apply pressure to the injection site for about 5 minutes.

- Never reinject the medication once you have made the initial injection, even if you fear that you have not injected yourself properly.

- Alternate sides with each injection.

- Do not inject medication more frequently than every 48–72 hours.

- If your erection lasts longer than 3 hours, call the urologist on call. Do not wait—a delay in seeking care will just make it more difficult to treat the prolonged erection.

- If you are having troubles with performing the injections, talk with your urologist. Perhaps getting more instructions or an auto-injector (e.g., the Pen-Inject 2.25 auto-injector) or teaching your partner would be helpful.

- Remember that with Edex and Caverject, once the medication has been reconstituted (i.e., once the powder is dissolved in the sterile water), it must be refrigerated. The solutions tend to lose their efficacy after 7 days.

Table 6   Dosage and Volume Calculations for Injection Therapy Using Prostaglandin E1 (Caverject, Edex)

10 µg/mL vial	Dose Volume 20 µg/mL vial	40 µg/mL vial
1.0 µg/0.10 mL	2.5 µg/0.125 mL	10 µg/0.25 mL
2.0 µg/0.20 mL	5.0 µg/0.25 mL	16 µg/0.40 mL
2.5 µg/0.25 mL	7.5 µg/0.375 mL	20 µg/0.50 mL
5.0 µg/0.50 mL	10.0 µg/0.50 mL	24 µg/0.6 mL
7.5 µg/0.75 mL	15.0 µg/0.75 mL	30 µg/0.75 mL
10.0 µg/1.0 mL	20 µg/1.0 mL	40 µg/1.0 mL

- Make sure that the volume of the medication and the dose of medication that you are injecting are consistent (see the calculation tables below).

- Do not reuse needles, and carefully dispose of used needles.

- Remember that your erection may persist after you climax and ejaculate, but will go down when the medication wears off and exits from your system.

58. What is the success rate of penile injection therapy?

Success rates for intracavernous injection therapy range from 70–94%. This kind of treatment is helpful in erectile dysfunction of all causes. Although injection therapy does not interfere with orgasm or ejaculation, its long-term success requires that the individual be comfortable with the injection process. Besides its

Intracavernous injection therapy is helpful in erectile dysfunction of all causes. Its long-term success requires that the individual be comfortable with the injection process.

overall success rate, another advantage of injection therapy is its quick onset of action, within 5 to 20 minutes of injection.

The dose required to achieve a successful erection varies greatly with the cause of the erectile dysfunction. Young men with spinal cord injury may require only 1 µg of Caverject or Edex, whereas older men with vascular disease and diabetes may require 40 µg of these medications.

In studies that compared injection therapy with other treatments for erectile dysfunction, injection therapy was found to be more effective than MUSE (alprostadil inserted into the urethra) in patients with erectile dysfunction. In addition, patients preferred injection therapy to MUSE, despite the need for injection, which most likely reflects the superior efficacy of injection therapy.

Injection therapy appears to be efficacious in men who have not responded to sildenafil (Viagra), an orally administered therapy. Because this therapy does not depend on the presence of intact nerves, patients with a neurologic component to their erectile dysfunction (i.e., those who have undergone non–nerve-sparing radical prostatectomies) often respond to injection therapy.

59. What are the risks of penile injection therapy?

Low Compliance

Despite the high efficacy and relatively benign side-effect profile of injection therapy, there is a high discontinuation rate with this treatment for erectile dysfunction. A recent review demonstrated that 15% of men who are offered injection therapy do not even try it, 40% discontinue treatment within 3 months, and only 20–30% of men continue with injection therapy for more than 3 years. Reasons for discontinuation include fear of needles, the injected volume, adverse effects, partner discontent with this mode of therapy, loss of partner or relationship issues, problems with the ability to administer the medication, and the return of spontaneous erections.

Pain

Approximately 30% of men have pain with injection therapy. This pain may consist of either injection site pain or, with Caverject or Edex, a diffuse penile pain. Men who experience penile pain with Caverject or Edex can be switched to triple P (prostaglandin E_1, phentolamine, and papaverine), which has a much lower incidence of penile pain.

Hematoma

Hematoma

A blister-like collection of blood under the skin.

If you do not look closely where you are injecting, it is possible to injure a superficial vein in the penis, causing a bruise, and, less frequently, a **hematoma** (a collection of blood). If this occurs, gentle pressure on the injection site will prevent further bleeding. The bruise or hematoma will resolve with time. Men taking blood thinners should be cautious when injecting medication and should always apply pressure after the injection is complete. If you experience significant penile swelling, you should contact your urologist.

Priapism

The risk of priapism with injection therapy is about 2%, and most of these cases occur during the initial test dosing. Triple P carries a higher risk of priapism than Caverject and Edex. If your erection lasts longer than 3 hours, you should contact your urologist or the urologist on call. Never re-inject the medication after you have initially injected it, no matter how little volume you think you received with the first injection. Do not combine therapies for erectile dysfunction without the prior approval and guidance of your urologist.

Penile Fibrosis

The development of scar tissue within the corpora is a risk of injection therapy, and this risk is higher with triple P than with Caverject and Edex. Over time, this problem may be manifested as a need to use a higher dose of medication to achieve an adequate erection.

Plaque Formation

One of the concerns with injection therapy is that each time the small needle pierces the tunica albuginea to enter the corpora, it causes minor trauma to the area. Theoretically, this trauma may cause plaques to form, as occurs in Peyronie's disease (see Question 31). Given this potential risk, men should not inject any more frequently than every 48 hours and should alternate sides. This will evenly distribute the trauma and keep the man's penis from curving to one side.

Liver Toxicity

The risk of liver injury with injection therapy is low and does not appear to be a concern for men taking Caverject or Edex. Liver function tests (blood tests obtained to assess how the liver is working) have shown elevated liver enzyme levels in men with a history of alcohol abuse or liver damage who were using intracavernous papaverine or papaverine in combination with phentolamine

Treatment

(bimix). Periodic liver function tests should be considered only in this patient subpopulation.

60. What is the vacuum device?

The vacuum device is a safe, reliable, reversible, noninvasive method of achieving an erection. The concept of treating erectile dysfunction by creating a negative pressure to "pull blood into the penis" was first described in 1874, but it was not until 1974 that Osbon developed the first commercially available vacuum device for this purpose. Although this device did not receive FDA approval until 1982, by 1990 it was one of the most commonly recommended therapies for erectile dysfunction. Many vacuum devices are on the market, all of which use essentially the same technique but vary in their method of inducing the vacuum and the types of constricting bands used. Purchasing a vacuum device requires a prescription. A variety of companies manufacture vacuum devices beside Osbon (which is now Timm), including Encore, Mentor Urology, Post-T-Vac, and Synergist. Caution should be exercised in the purchase and use of similar devices advertised in magazines as sex aids because these devices may not have built-in pressure valves and may cause harm.

The function of the device is based on two principles:

1. A vacuum, or negative pressure, is generated to pull blood into the penis.

2. A constriction device (ring) is used at the base of the penis to decrease venous drainage and thus prolong the erection.

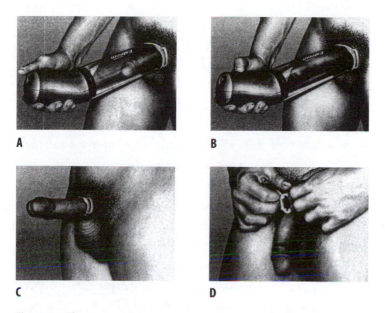

A   B

C   D

Figure 9   The vacuum device. (A) The vacuum device's pump creates a suction that pulls blood into the penis. (B) Within minutes, a nearly natural erection is produced. (C) A band is placed at the base of the penis to hold blood in the penis. (D) The constructing band is removed after intercourse. It should not be left on for more than 30 minutes. Reprinted with permission from Timm Medical Technologies, Inc.

The vacuum device consists of a plastic cylinder, a pump that is either battery or hand operated, and one or more constrictive bands (Figure 9). The cylinder is wide enough and long enough to accommodate the erect penis. It is closed at the tip and open at the base. The constrictive bands are preloaded onto the base of the cylinder before its use.

Bob's comment:

I have tried the vacuum device but never had much satisfaction with it. For me, the preparation and the mechanics of achieving and sustaining an erection with the device were too much. I was dubious right from the onset, when the vacuum device's manufacturer's representative met with me in the doctor's office to demonstrate the device. He unveiled a 10-inch cylindrical container that was placed over my flaccid penis after I had affixed some Mason jar-type rubber rings at the base of the device. After the vacuum device had created an erection, I would have to dislodge these rings from the base of the device so that they were around the base of my penis. The rings would then squeeze the base of my penis to maintain the erection.

My skepticism started the day that the representative showed me the device and assisted me with a live demonstration, at which time I asked myself, "Who designed this thing?" In fact, I really questioned why the representative would want this job—surely there were other career opportunities that he found more appealing. My skepticism persisted because despite the arduous presexual preparation, the vacuum device just never worked adequately for me. The rubber rings didn't seem to be sufficiently tight to maintain the erection. I will say, however, that of all of the other therapies that I tried before the placement of a penile prosthesis, the vacuum device did produce the firmest erection.

Perhaps it was my attitude; maybe it was my physiology. However, even though I used the vacuum device a score of times over a year or so, I knew that this was not for me over the long term. The romanticism and the spontaneity of sex were not there with the vacuum device.

61. Who is a candidate for the vacuum device?

Most men may use the vacuum device, and there are relatively few contraindications to its use. Men who have bleeding problems or who are taking blood thinners can use the vacuum device but must be careful. Men with Peyronie's disease who have significant penile curvature may not be able to use the device because the erect penis may not fit in the cylinder. In such cases, corrective surgery to straighten the penis may be performed before the use of the vacuum device, or the man can try using the device and generating a less rigid erection. An uncooperative partner precludes the successful use of the device.

62. How do I use the vacuum device?

To use the vacuum device, the constricting band is first placed onto the base of the cylinder, and the cylinder is then placed over the penis and pressed firmly against the pubic bone to achieve an airtight seal (Figure 9). Suction is applied by either a battery- or hand-operated pump. When the penis is rigid, the band is slipped off the cylinder and onto the base of the penis. When intercourse is finished, the band is removed, and the blood drains out of the penis.

The time taken to achieve an erection with the vacuum device varies but may be as short as 2–3 minutes. The band may be left on the penis for 30 minutes only. Most men are able to quickly learn how to use the device and become comfortable with using it within four practice sessions.

63. What are the success and satisfaction rates for the vacuum device?

The initial report on the vacuum device, which was published in 1985, reported a 90% success rate for this device in achieving an erection that was adequate for sexual performance. Since then, published success rates (i.e., the ability to have a rigid erection) with the vacuum device have ranged from 84–95%, and overall satisfaction rates reported for this device have ranged from 72–94%. Notably, the vacuum device has been shown to be effective in treating men with erectile dysfunction of many different causes. In patients with spinal cord injuries, the success rate is reported to be 92%. In those with psychogenic erectile dysfunction, this device also yields good results. In men who have erectile dysfunction caused by arterial disease or after radical prostatectomy, the success rate ranges from 90–100%. Furthermore, the vacuum device is successful in some men who were impotent after the removal of a penile prosthesis.

Approximately 50–70% of individuals continue to use the vacuum device over the long term. Reasons for discontinuation of this therapy include issues unrelated to the device (e.g., return of spontaneous erections, loss of libido, or loss of partner), which were cited in 43% of cases in one study. In 57% of cases, the reason for discontinuation is related to side effects of the device or partner dissatisfaction.

Several studies have compared the vacuum device with other forms of treatment for erectile dysfunction. In a study of men who were using the vacuum device successfully and then tried sildenafil (Viagra), approximately one third preferred to resume use of the vacuum device rather than continue with the oral medication, citing the fact that the vacuum device gave them a better-quality erection. In a study that compared intracavernosal therapy (injection therapy) with the vacuum device, there was a trend among younger patients who had a shorter period of erectile dysfunction to favor intracavernosal therapy.

Bob's comment:

I did not have very good results with this device. However, many users have achieved excellent results with this technology.

64. What are the side effects of the vacuum device?

Side effects of the vacuum device include the following:

- Penile coolness. With the vacuum device, penile skin temperature may decrease by 18°C.

- Penile skin cyanosis. Congestion outside the corpora may make the penile skin look blue. This problem resolves with removal of the constricting band.

- Increased girth. The penile width after use of the vacuum device is actually wider than is seen with a normal erection.

- Pain. The most common complaint, pain usually occurs when men first use the device. It may be related to either the vacuum or the constricting band. Discomfort during suction is noted in 20–40% of men who use the vacuum device, primarily in men who are just learning to use the device. The pain appears to decrease with continued use of the vacuum device and may be related to initial unfamiliarity with the device. As many as 45% of men have pain at the site of the constricting band. Again, this discomfort seems to improve with time and familiarity with the device.

Complication

An undesirable result of a treatment, surgery, or medication.

Ischemia

A deficiency of blood flow to an area that compromises the health of the tissue.

Prosthesis

An artificial device used to replace the lost normal function of a structure or organ in the body.

- Ejaculatory troubles. Pain with ejaculation is reported by 3–15% of men who use the vacuum device, and inability to ejaculate occurs in 12–30%.

- Penile bruising. This side effect is noted in 6–20% of men who use the vacuum device.

- Numbness during erection. This side effect occurs in 5% of men who use the vacuum device.

- Partner dissatisfaction. This rate ranges from 6–11%, with the following reasons for dissatisfaction being cited: unhappy with the performance, penile temperature, and penile appearance.

Severe **complications** (serious, undesired results of a treatment) are uncommon with use of the vacuum device, but they can occur. In particular, ischemia (decreased blood flow) of the penis leading to necrosis can occur if the constricting band is left on too long. This complication is more of a problem in men with spinal cord injuries because they do not feel the discomfort related to the band. If the band is removed within 30 minutes of application, the risk of penile **ischemia** is rare.

65. What is a penile prosthesis?

A penile **prosthesis** is an artificial device that, when placed in the penis, allows a man to have an erection. The development and use of penile prostheses began in the 1970s. Since then, numerous revisions and modifications in the prostheses have improved the satisfaction rate and mechanical durability of these devices.

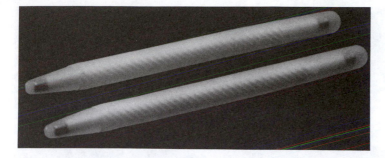

Figure 10   One piece, semi-rigid penile prosthesis. Reprinted with permission from American Medical Systems.

The first prosthesis developed was a "rigid" prosthesis. With this device, a rigid cylinder was placed into each of the corpora cavernosa. Each cylinder had a fixed length and girth and remained "erect" at all times. The limiting factor was the inability to conceal one's penis.

The next type of prosthesis developed was the "semirigid" prosthesis (Figure 10). Its cylinder contains a flexible metal coil in the center that is surrounded by silicone. Like the rigid prosthesis, the semirigid prosthesis also has a fixed length and girth; unlike the rigid prosthesis, it can be bent down to provide for concealment.

The most commonly used prostheses are inflatable models, which vary from self-contained inflatable prostheses to multipart inflatable prostheses. American Medical Systems makes an inflatable prosthesis that consists of only two cylinders (Figure 10) that contain a pump at their tips. When placed into the corpora of the penis, the pump lies in the glans. Gentle squeezing of the glans activates the pump, which transfers fluid from one compartment of the cylinder to another. This fluid transfer creates the rigidity needed for an erection. To deflate the prosthesis, the penis is bent over one's hand with gentle pressure on the corpora, which

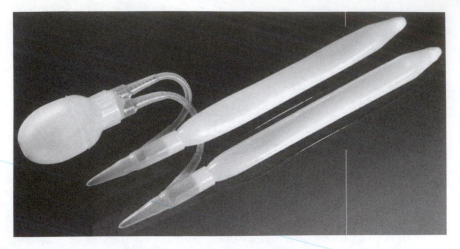

Figure 11   Two-piece penile prosthesis. The two long cylinders are surgically inserted into the corpora, while the pump/reservoir in the center is palced in the scrotum.

drains the fluid back into the other compartment of the cylinder. Although a self-contained inflatable prosthesis is simple to use, the main drawback is that it can provide only limited girth.

More popular than the self-contained models are the multipart inflatable prostheses, of which there are two types: two-piece units, which consist of two cylinders and a combined pump and reservoir in the scrotum (Figure 11), and three-piece units, which comprise two cylinders, a scrotal pump, and a separate reservoir that is placed in the pelvis (Figure 12). The advantage of the three-piece unit is that it allows for the maximal amount of fluid transfer given the larger reservoir size. Also, when placed correctly, the device and its tubing are completely concealed, so one is able to void in the locker room without anyone knowing that the multipart prosthesis is present. Multipart inflatable prostheses are made by two companies, American Medical Systems and Mentor Urology.

Treatment

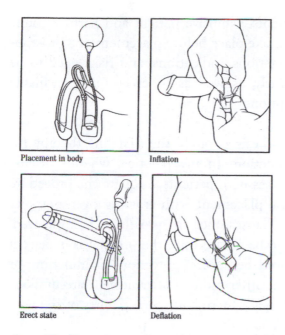

Placement in body

Inflation

Erect state

Deflation

Figure 12   Three-piece penile prosthesis. Drawings of the AMS 700CX™/CXM™ Penile Prosthesis courtesy of American Medical Systems, Inc., Minnetonka, Minnesota (www.visitAMS.com).

Placement of a penile prosthesis requires extensive patient and partner discussion. It is not considered a first-line therapy in most cases of erectile dysfunction, but is an appropriate therapy for well-counseled individuals who have not responded to other therapies or who have found those alternatives to be unsatisfactory.

66. Who is a candidate for a penile prosthesis?

Penile prostheses are usually placed in men with organic erectile dysfunction. In men with psychogenic erectile dysfunction, extensive counseling should be administered and other treatment options should be exhausted before a penile prosthesis is considered. For all other patients, extensive patient and partner counseling should take place before placement of a prosthesis; the expectations, indications, and risks need to be discussed clearly, as well as other currently available and future options.

A penile prosthesis is not considered a first-line therapy in most cases of erectile dysfunction, but is an appropriate therapy for well-counseled individuals who have not responded to other therapies or who have found those alternatives to be unsatisfactory.

A penile prosthesis is rarely the first-line therapy for erectile dysfunction. In my practice, when I discuss penile prostheses with patients, I equate the procedure for its surgical placement with crossing over a rickety bridge that collapses once the prosthesis is implanted. You cannot go backward once the prosthesis is placed; if it is removed because of infection, malfunction, or dissatisfaction, other options of treatment are unlikely to work. Although there have been reports of the vacuum device and injection therapy working in some individuals after removal of a prosthesis, these instances are not common. For all these reasons, it is best to try all available therapies and determine whether they are successful and satisfactory before placement of a prosthesis occurs.

Indications for a penile prosthesis include the following:

- The patient's unwillingness to consider, failure to respond to, or inability to continue with other forms of treatment, such as oral therapy, injection therapy, MUSE, and the vacuum device

- Postinjection therapy penile fibrosis

- Peyronie's disease and erectile dysfunction

- Postpriapism erectile dysfunction

- Sex-change operations in women who undergo surgical creation of a penis

- Penile amputations in men, who then undergo surgical creation of a penis

- Psychogenic erectile dysfunction, after extensive counseling and evaluation

- Neurogenic bladders requiring condom catheters for urinary drainage

67. How do I use the penile prosthesis, and how is it placed?

Placement of a penile prosthesis is a surgical procedure that can be performed under general anesthesia (an unconscious state in which the patient does not feel any pain) or spinal anesthesia (anesthesia produced by injection of a local anesthetic into the subarachnoid space around the spinal cord). You will stay in the hospital overnight (i.e., you have an **inpatient** stay) and are usually able to go home the following morning.

To minimize the risk of infection, prior to the procedure your scrotal area is shaved and you are scrubbed with an antibacterial soap for 10–15 minutes. In addition, you are given intravenous antibiotics to kill any residual bacteria that may be present on your skin. These intravenous antibiotics will be continued during your entire hospital stay, and you are discharged to home with a 10- to 14-day supply of oral antibiotics.

Once you are asleep or your spinal anesthesia is functioning, you are shaved and prepped. A **Foley catheter**

Inpatient

A patient who is admitted to the hospital for treatment.

Foley catheter

A catheter that is placed into the bladder via the urethra to drain urine.

is placed through your penis and into your bladder to empty the bladder and to allow for identification of the urethra, the tube you urinate through (which has the catheter in it), so as to prevent injury to it during the surgery.

Three approaches to placement of the penile prosthesis are used, and the location of the incision varies with the type of prosthesis being placed and your surgeon's preference:

1. A *subcoronal incision,* a circumcision-type incision, is used for placement of semirigid prostheses.

2. A *penoscrotal incision* is used for placement of multi-part prostheses, for reoperations, and in cases of penile fibrosis (scarring). This kind of incision is made in the midline of the upper part of the scrotum. If you look at your scrotum, you will see that a line runs up the middle of the scrotum; the incision is made in this line so that when it heals, it will be incorporated in the normal scrotal line.

3. Some surgeons use an *infrapubic incision* for placement of multipart prostheses. This kind of incision is made below the pubic bone near the base of the penis.

Usually, all components of a multipart prosthesis can be placed through a single incision. In some patients, prior abdominal and groin surgery—such as a hernia repair or a radical prostatectomy—may make placement of the reservoir of the three-piece prosthesis difficult. In this situation, your surgeon may make another incision on your abdomen to enable the reservoir to be implanted correctly. Each corpora cavernosa is opened and dilated to accommodate the cylinder. Each corpora is then measured. Your penis is actually much longer than you think—it extends back behind your pubic bone—and it is very important that the correct size of cylinder be placed. The pump is implanted either in the midline of your scrotum between the two testicles or on one side of the scrotum. You should discuss pump placement with your surgeon before surgery to ensure that its location will be easy for you to maneuver, particularly if you do not have good use of both hands.

It is important that the corpora are fully dilated and that appropriate-length cylinders are selected. If the cylinders are too long, they may cause discomfort during intercourse. If the cylinders are too short, they will not provide adequate support to the tip of the penis, causing the glans to droop. This drooping of the glans may make it difficult to perform vaginal penetration. Such a glans droop can be corrected by a simple surgical procedure and often does not require replacement of the prosthesis.

The reservoir in the three-piece unit is placed in the pelvis near the bladder. The tubing that connects the reservoir, pump, and cylinders runs deep under your skin so that it is not visible; if you feel closely, you may be able to identify the tubing, but the goal is to have it be unnoticeable. Before the procedure is completed, your surgeon will test the prosthesis to ensure that all components are working well, that when inflated it gives you a fully rigid erection, and that the tips of the prosthesis are in a good position in the tip of your penis.

Before the incision is closed, a small drain is placed to prevent a hematoma (collection of blood) from forming, and the prosthesis is deflated. The surgeon may leave the prosthesis partially inflated and then deflate it the following morning; this step can sometimes help prevent bleeding. When you wake up from surgery in the recovery room, you will have a catheter in place that drains your urine; a dressing around your penis, which will be taped up against your abdomen; and a drain in place.

In men with erectile dysfunction and prostate cancer who are undergoing a radical prostatectomy for treatment of their prostate cancer, the prosthesis can be placed at the time of surgery. There does not appear to be an increased risk of infection when this route is taken.

Bob's comment:

[I had my penile prosthesis] placed under general anesthesia. I will discuss the hospital and postoperative course in [Question 68].

As part of the initial discussion on the penile prosthesis, Dr. Ellsworth discussed the mechanics of the prosthesis with me. As she was explaining the mechanics of the prosthesis, she must have noticed a puzzled look on my part. She said, "Do you want to see one?" "Sure," I responded. She returned carrying a rubbery device that had a manually operated pump at one end with two tentacles approximately 7 or 8 inches long protruding from either side. Frankly, it reminded me of one of those Day-Glo plastic Halloween skeletons that bobble all over the place. I said (to myself this time), "Is that thing going into my body?" It was. Incidentally, Dr. Ellsworth urged me to take the device home (in a brown paper bag) to show my wife and familiarize ourselves with the device.

After placement of the prosthesis and my hospital stay, . . . I wanted nothing to do with activating the device for the first 3–4 weeks because of soreness in the vicinity of the incision. During this time, Dr. Ellsworth examined me periodically to ensure that there were no signs of a dreaded bacterial infection. Finally, when the tenderness had abated, the time came for Dr. Ellsworth to demonstrate how the penile prosthesis worked. The pump—the part that produces the erection—is inside the scrotum. It is somewhat rectangular in shape, about the size of a caramel candy, with a ball-type pump affixed on one side and the release valves along either end of the device. In principle, it works this way: Before intercourse, one locates the pump and presses it six or seven times to transfer fluid from the reservoir into the penile cylinders to create an erection. The penis will remain rigid as long as one desires. When one is finished with intercourse, one squeezes the release valves, and the fluid drains out of the cylinders and back into the reservoir. Gentle squeezing on the penis helps to get all of the fluid out of the cylinders. As with anything new, it is difficult to use initially, but with practice, it becomes much easier to use. It is not long before you adapt. It merely becomes part of you.

68. What are the hospital course and the postoperative course like with placement of a penile prosthesis?

The morning after surgery, the drain and the catheter will be removed. You will be instructed about taping your penis to your abdomen. If the prosthesis was left partially inflated, it will be deflated and should remain

Autoinflation

Pertaining to a penile prosthesis, the spontaneous inflation of the prosthesis without manual pumping.

If the prosthesis "autoinflates" during the first month after the surgery, such that you have a partial erection without using the pump, you should call your surgeon and arrange to have the device deflated.

deflated during the first month after surgery. During the first month after the surgery, the prosthesis may sometimes **"autoinflate,"** such that you will note that you have a partial erection without using the pump. If this occurs, you should call your surgeon and arrange to have the device deflated. During this time of healing, your body "walls off" the prosthesis. It does not consider the prosthesis to be part of your normal body, so it produces a tissue layer around the prosthesis. It is important that this tissue layer (called a capsule) forms around a full reservoir so that autoinflation will not be a long-term problem.

You will be discharged to home after you have voided at the hospital. At the time of your discharge, you will receive prescriptions for antibiotics and pain medications. You can shower roughly 3 days after your surgery and tub bathe in 1 week. You will be seen periodically during the first month after your surgery to ensure that all is healing well and that there are no signs of infection. You should contact your physician if you note any increasing pain, swelling, drainage from your incision, or fever during this time.

After the healing is complete and you are comfortable, you will be taught how to use your prosthesis. This appointment usually occurs 4–6 weeks after the initial surgery. Do not be surprised if you find it difficult to use the prosthesis at first. It is often helpful to bring your partner with you to this instructional visit so that the two of you can work on figuring it out together. Your surgeon may also provide movies and instructional booklets to assist you in learning how the prosthesis functions. I find that letting men take a sample prosthesis home with them is helpful in getting to know its workings better. Do not get discouraged—if you are having trouble working with the prosthesis, call your surgeon. All it takes is more education and more practice.

Bob's comment:

I arrived at the hospital early in the morning. Although I anticipated a few snickers from the hospital staff because of the nature of the procedure, I encountered only professionalism from the entire hospital staff, from admission through discharge.

I was placed in a hospital bed in the same-day surgery area, dressed in a hospital gown, and hooked up to intravenous fluids. I quickly succumbed to a sedative that I was given before the surgery, and suddenly when I awoke, I was in a hospital bed in the hospital room. The procedure was over. I had been out for about 4 hours, in which time I had been prepped, implanted, and returned to a hospital room.

Upon regaining consciousness, I immediately sensed that I had undergone the surgery because of soreness emanating from my scrotum whenever I moved. Exploring, I put my hand on my penis. A bandage covered the area, and I could feel a rather large incision in the area of my testicles. Dr. Ellsworth stopped by to assure me that everything had gone well but that she was concerned about infection, particularly given that I was a diabetic, and that if infection occurred it would require removal of the implant and a repeat procedure at another time in the future. Ugh! I had to make sure that no bacterial germs descended on me.

About that time, I noticed that I had a roommate. At Dartmouth–Hitchcock Medical Center, patients are rather arbitrarily assigned to a private or semiprivate room based on availability. Just my luck—no private rooms were available. Even in my semicomatose condition, I knew instinctively that I was not going to share the reason for my "operation" with my roommate. Deviously, I prepared myself for the inevitable question, "What did you have done?" I learned that my roomie, a 30-year-old man from Vermont, was recovering from surgery on his leg because of a "real" injury from an earlier farm accident. I responded to the "inevitable" question, telling him that I had surgery on a groin muscle that I had injured. How pleased I was with the near-accurate deception. After all, how could I admit to an enhancement of my penis? Not macho!

The floor nurses were very helpful throughout my overnight stay. Painkiller medications and a sleeping pill helped me pass the night. Never once did anyone imply that the surgery was cosmetic or vanity induced. My male nurse confided in me that I was the first patient that he had assisted who had undergone an implant.

Dr. Ellsworth came by the following morning, checked my incision, removed the drain, and said that she was happy with my progress and that I was able to go home. The catheter was removed, and I promptly voided on my own. I said goodbye to my roommate, who I overheard earlier telling his wife, to my satisfaction, that I had had "ligament surgery."

Dr. Ellsworth advised me at discharge that I would feel somewhat awkward for about 30 days. I was instructed to cleanse my incision with hydrogen peroxide and to apply an antibiotic ointment to the incision. I was to keep my penis secured to my abdomen until the first postoperative visit. The ordeal was over. I headed home, fully implanted.

69. What is the success rate of the penile prosthesis?

In well-counseled individuals, the success/satisfaction rate with the penile prosthesis ranges from 80–91%. Partner satisfaction rates have been reported to range from 70–90%. In fact, in one study, 92% of patients and 90% of partners indicated that they would choose the implant surgery if faced with the option again.

Bob's comment:

As a lay person who has undergone placement of a penile prosthesis for erectile dysfunction, I see the advantages of the prosthesis to be as follows:

- *One can have an erection as long as one would like without worry.*

- *[The penile prosthesis] does not rely on drugs or chemicals.*

- *After some initial getting used to it, the implant is fairly easy to use and can be activated quickly and unobtrusively.*

- *It is permanent.*

- *It works when other therapies fail.*

- *Being able to participate in intercourse has a positive impact on one's self-image—it is a good feeling to know that you are capable of resuming and enjoying the full intimacies of your relationship with your partner again.*

Treatment

70. What are the risks and complications of a penile prosthesis?

As with any surgical procedure, there are complications associated with the placement of a penile prosthesis. These risks may be subdivided into intraoperative complications (those occurring during surgery) and postoperative complications (those occurring after surgery).

Intraoperative (During Surgery) Complications

Perforation

During dilation of the corpora cavernosa, the dilating instrument can perforate the urethra. If this occurs, the procedure must be terminated, the catheter must be left in place, and the urethra must be allowed to heal. If one cylinder has already been placed on the other side, it may be left in place and connected to the pump and reservoir before the surgery is completed. If the patient desires, the surgeon can go back in a few months and try to replace the cylinder. Some men find that they are able to achieve adequate rigidity with only one cylinder in place and do not wish to undergo another surgical procedure.

Similarly, during dilation of the corpora, a hole may be made from one corpus cavernosum into the other. The surgery can continue in this case, but the cylinders must be properly placed in each corpus cavernosum. If a hole is made, a cylinder may cross over, meaning that it starts in one corpus cavernosum but passes through the hole and ends in the other corpus cavernosum. If this situation goes unrecognized, it may cause asymmetry and pain with use of the prosthesis.

Existing Scarring

In individuals with significant penile fibrosis, such severe scarring may be present that narrower cylinders will be required. Rarely, it will be difficult to close the corpora over the cylinders. A patch of synthetic material or tissue must be removed from another area of your body in this case and used to cover the corporal defect.

Residual Curvature of the Penis

In patients with Peyronie's disease, placement of the prosthesis and maneuvering of the prosthesis when it is erect in the operating room are usually all that is needed to correct the penile curvature. On rare occasions, residual curvature may be observed after placement of the prosthesis. If this does not improve with use of the prosthesis, then another procedure may be performed to excise the plaque.

Excessive Bleeding and Anesthesia Complications

As with all surgical procedures, there are bleeding and anesthetic risks with the implantation of a penile prosthesis.

Postoperative (After-Surgery) Complications

Decreased Penile Length

Decreased penile length is actually not a complication of penile implantation, but rather is intrinsic to the surgery. The cylinders are of a fixed length. To obtain penile rigidity, the cylinders increase in width (girth). Very observant patients will note a 1- to 2-cm decrease in penile length after the procedure.

Infection

One of the most devastating complications of penile prosthesis surgery is infection. Infection rates range from 2–16% in first-time procedures but increase to 8–18% in reoperations. Patients with diabetes and spinal cord injury, in particular, are at increased risk for infection.

Erosion

Destruction of a tissue surface—for example a penile prosthesis eroding through the skin.

Signs of infection include persistent pain, **erosion** of a part of the prosthesis, purulent drainage, fever, swelling and redness of the scrotum, and fixation of the tubing to the scrotal skin. In most cases, but particularly when infection occurs early after implantation, the entire prosthesis must be removed emergently. The area must then be irrigated with antibiotics, and intravenous antibiotics followed by oral antibiotics must be given. Implantation of a second prosthesis can be attempted 6 months later, after the area has completely healed.

Salvage

A procedure intended to "rescue" a patient who has failed to respond to a prior therapy.

When an infection occurs later and is caused by less aggressive bacteria, the surgeon may try to **salvage** (rescue or save) the prosthesis. In such a case, the patient is taken to the operating room, the infected prosthesis is removed, the area is irrigated copiously with antibiotic solutions, and a new prosthesis is placed. The risk of infection associated with the new prosthesis in this situation is about 15%.

Erosion and Migration

Migration

Spontaneous change of place.

Erosion (destruction of a tissue surface) and **migration** (spontaneous change of place) of the prosthesis occur more commonly with placement of rigid prostheses and in men with indwelling catheters or on clean intermittent catheterization. These complications may also occur when the prosthesis is too long or the patient has an unsuspected urethral injury.

In the case of urethral erosion, there may be some splaying of the urine stream and the tip of the prosthesis may protrude into the urethra. In such cases, the affected cylinder is removed, and the corpora are irrigated with an antibiotic solution and closed. A catheter is placed into the bladder for about 1 week to promote urethral healing. A new cylinder can be placed 6 months later.

The tubing may also erode through the skin. Such tubing erosion is often a sign of a smoldering infection, in which case the best thing to do is to remove the prosthesis. The surgeon can also attempt the salvage technique described earlier.

Lastly, the cylinders may migrate proximally toward the base of the penis, a condition that shows up as a new droop in the glans. When this happens, the cylinder must be removed, the defect in the corpus cavernosum corrected, and the cylinder replaced.

Glans Droop

If the cylinders to be implanted are too short, they will not provide adequate support to the tip of the penis, causing the glans to droop. This drooping of the glans may make it difficult for the man to achieve vaginal penetration. A glans droop can be corrected by a simple surgical procedure and often does not require replacement of the prosthesis.

Penile Ischemia and Necrosis

These complications, which are extremely rare, occur when there is an injury to the blood supply to the corpora cavernosa or to the glans. Men with severe diabetes, those with extensive vascular disease, and those who require an extensive dissection for placement of the prosthesis are at increased risk of developing penile ischemia or necrosis. If the postoperative dressing is too tight, it may also cause ischemia.

Perineal Pain

Patients often experience some discomfort during the first 2 months or so after placement of a penile prosthesis. If the pain persists for a longer period, your physician may evaluate whether you have an infection or whether the prosthesis is too large. Some men may experience penile discomfort with the initial inflation of the prosthesis that is related to stretching of the tunica (the thick white membrane wrapped around the corpora cavernosa), but this usually resolves with time as the tunica stretches.

Residual Penile Curvature

In patients with Peyronie's disease, placement of the prosthesis and maneuvering of the prosthesis when it is erect in the operating room are usually all that is needed to correct the penile curvature that can occur with this condition. In rare cases, residual curvature may persist after placement of the prosthesis. If this condition does not improve with use of the prosthesis, then another procedure may be performed to excise the plaque.

Mechanical Problems

The incidence of mechanical problems with prostheses is approximately 5%—quite a low rate. Such problems may potentially include leaks, aneurysms, and rupture of the cylinders.

Leaks typically occur at connection sites and where the cylinder tubing enters the cylinder. Leaking prostheses either will not work or will not provide adequate rigidity. Connection site leaks may be easily repaired. A leaking cylinder can be replaced, but it is recommended that the entire prosthesis be replaced if the prosthesis has been implanted for a few years.

Aneurysms (i.e., dilations of a part of the cylinder) are very uncommon with the current prosthesis models. If they occur, the affected cylinder must be removed and replaced with a new device.

The cylinders can also rupture, usually as a result of unrecognized damage during the closure of the corpora. This problem is often detected when the device is inflated 4 to 6 weeks after surgery.

Autoinflation

Autoinflation is the phenomenon whereby the device inflates on its own without you manipulating the pump. It is the result of increased pressure around the reservoir. Autoinflation may occur intermittently during the first month after placement of the prosthesis but should not occur thereafter. It is important during the first month after the implantation of the device to deflate the prosthesis quickly to prevent persistence of the autoinflation. If an adequate space was not created for the reservoir at the time of surgery, the autoinflation will not resolve, and an additional procedure will be required to correct the problem.

Bob's comment:

As I think about the penile prosthesis and the surgery, I see the disadvantages of the prosthesis to be as follows:

Treatment

Aneurysm

Pertaining to a penile prosthesis, an abnormal dilation of the prosthesis related to weakening of a part of the cylinder.

- *The dreaded risk of infection [is a major concern].*

- *The procedure requires a surgical intervention and a night's stay in the hospital, which is expensive.*

- *If one examines the penis closely, one can feel the tubing and cylinders.*

71. What is penile bypass surgery, and who is a candidate?

The goal in penile bypass surgery is to increase blood flow to the penis so that spontaneous erections can occur. Because of the technical complexity of this surgery, few men are actually candidates for it. The ideal candidate is a healthy man who has a discrete arterial narrowing and no known medical conditions (e.g., diabetes mellitus, hypertension, elevated cholesterol level, and cardiovascular disease) that might potentially complicate future arterial function.

The aim of penile bypass surgery is to provide an alternative arterial pathway that does not rely on the obstructed artery.

72. Who performs penile bypass surgery, and how is it done?

The surgery is typically performed by a urologist who specializes in the treatment of erectile dysfunction. The urologist may also work with a vascular surgeon—that is, a surgeon who performs bypass procedures to treat blood flow problems throughout the body. This highly technical procedure should be performed by

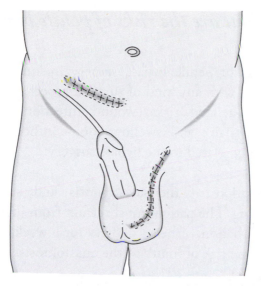

Figure 13 **Incisions for penile bypass surgery. Adapted with permission from Carson C, Kirby R, Goldstein I. Textbook of Erectile Dysfunction. Oxford, UK: Isis Medical Medical Media, 1999, p. 404.**

surgeons who are experienced with this type of surgery. Your local urologist may refer you to the appropriately trained surgeon in your area.

The penile bypass procedure may be performed under general or spinal anesthesia. Often, two incisions are made: one in the lower abdomen to provide access for the *donor artery* (the artery that will bring blood into the penis), and one in the opposite groin area to provide access for the *recipient artery* (the artery to which the donor artery will be sewn) (Figure 13).

73. What is the success rate of penile bypass surgery?

The reported success rates for penile bypass surgery range from 30–84%. Careful patient selection helps to optimize the long-term results.

74. What are the risks of penile bypass surgery?

The risks of penile bypass surgery include the risks associated with any kind of surgical procedure, such as anesthetic-related risks, wound infection, bleeding, incisional pain, and swelling. Some other risks are specifically related to the bypass surgery:

- Disruption of the anastomosis and subsequent bleeding. The patient must refrain from intercourse, masturbation, or heavy activity for 6 weeks to minimize the risk of injury to the anastomosis.

- Penile pain.

- Loss of penile sensation. This complication occurs as a result of trauma to the nerve that supplies sensation to the penis.

- Glans hyperemia—increased blood flow to the glans (tip) of the penis. This complication occurs in 7–13% of patients who undergo penile bypass surgery.

- Groin hernia.

- Thrombosis (obstruction) of the graft. If the blood flow through the graft is not adequate, then thrombosis (the formation of a clot) may occur in the graft.

75. What is venous ligation surgery?

Venous ligation surgery is a surgical procedure in which the veins that are responsible for the venous leak are identified and ligated (tied off). Cavernosometry (see Question 23) and cavernosography (see Question 24) are required before surgery to confirm the presence of a venous leak and to identify the site(s) of venous leak.

76. Who is a candidate for venous ligation surgery?

Men whose erectile dysfunction is caused by a venous leak are candidates for venous ligation surgery. In such cases, it is important to rule out other arterial disease that may be occurring along with the venous leak; therefore, these individuals should undergo an arterial assessment by color-flow Doppler ultrasound prior to their surgery. In addition, there should be no medical contraindications to surgery. Men who are interested in pursuing venous ligation surgery should be aware of the risks, benefits, success rates, and alternatives to this procedure.

77. What are the success rate and the risks of the venous ligation surgery?

Most patients who undergo venous ligation surgery for erectile dysfunction caused by venous leaks will notice immediate improvements in their erectile function after recovering from the surgery. Unfortunately, this effect appears to be lost over time, so that the long-term success rate for this procedure is only 50%. In men who do not respond over the long term, repeat cavernosography often demonstrates new sites of venous leak in these patients.

Complications and risks of the venous ligation surgery include the risks associated with any kind of surgical procedure, including anesthetic risks, infection, and bleeding. Complications and risks that are specific to venous ligation include prolonged penile swelling and failure to restore erectile function.

78. Who performs venous ligation surgery, and how is it done?

Not every institution in the United States is set up to accommodate venous ligation surgery. More precisely, most local urologists do not perform this surgery, but they should be able to give you the name and location of the closest urologist who does perform this procedure. Institutions that perform the surgery are also capable of conducting the specialized tests needed to confirm and localize the site(s) of venous leak—that is, cavernosometry and cavernosography. These tests must be carried out before venous ligation surgery is considered, and it is best to undergo these tests at the same institution where you plan to have the surgery.

The venous ligation procedure may be conducted under spinal or general anesthesia. The surgery is often performed through an inguinoscrotal incision (an incision that starts in your groin and extends down into your scrotum) and requires an extensive dissection of both the superficial and the deep penile veins. During the surgery, the veins responsible for the venous leak are tied off. Intraoperative studies can help delineate the sites of the leakage, and at the conclusion of the procedure, they can confirm that a rigid erection can be obtained and that there are no residual sites of venous leak.

79. What is apomorphine SL?

Apomorphine (Uprima) is a medication that has been used in the past to treat patients with Parkinson's disease. It works centrally (i.e., on the **central nervous system**) on the brain, causing the brain to increase the stimulation to the pelvic nerves. Apomorphine is not currently available in the United States, but it has been approved for use overseas. It is supplied as 2- and 3-mg sublingual (SL—placed under the tongue) tablets. This formulation has been investigated for erectile dysfunction because it produces a response similar to that obtained with other (non-SL) formulations of apomorphine but has fewer side effects. In addition, the SL route of administration ensures that the drug is absorbed quite quickly. Indeed, measurable blood levels of apomorphine are apparent within 10 minutes of the tablet's placement under the tongue, and peak levels occur 40–60 minutes after the drug is taken.

There does not appear to be any need to adjust the dose of apomorphine with older age. If you have renal or liver failure, you should take the lower dose (2 mg). You should use caution when using apomorphine if you also take antihypertensive medications (beta blockers, diuretics, or angiotensin-converting enzyme [ACE] inhibitors) or nitrate-containing medications (see Table 3, Question 45). The combination of apomorphine and an antihypertensive or nitrate may lower your blood pressure to unexpected levels. Similarly, if you consume large quantities of alcohol around the same time you take apomorphine, this combination may lower your blood pressure. It is recommended that no more than 0.3 mg/kg of alcohol be ingested around the time of apomorphine use. For the average 70-kg (155-pound) man, this would be the equivalent of a pint of beer, two glasses of wine, or two single measures of spirits. Also, if you experience postural or **orthostatic hypotension** (lowering of the blood pressure upon standing), you should use apomorphine SL with caution.

Central nervous system

The portion of the nervous system consisting of the brain and the spinal cord.

Apomorphine is not currently available in the United States, but it has been approved for use overseas.

Orthostatic hypotension

The acute lowering of blood pressure when a person changes from a sitting or lying position to an upright position (standing). Also called postural hypotension.

Treatment

Contraindications to the use of apomorphine include prior allergic reactions to this medication, severe unstable angina, recent myocardial infarction, severe heart failure, low blood pressure (hypotension), or other medical conditions in which sexual activity is not advisable.

80. How do I use apomorphine SL?

It is recommended that you start with 2 mg of apomorphine SL. If that dose is not effective and you have no contraindications to increasing the dose, you may switch to 3 mg of apomorphine SL, as your doctor prescribes. Apomorphine SL is a sublingual medication, meaning that the pill is placed under your tongue. As with sildenafil (Viagra), this medication is taken on demand, before anticipated sexual activity.

Apomorphine SL is not currently being produced in the United States, and it remains to be seen whether it will become available here in the future. It is currently available in Europe.

81. What is the success rate of apomorphine? What are the side effects?

Studies using both 2 and 3 mg of sublingual apomorphine have shown that this medication is more effective than placebo in producing erections that are firm enough for intercourse. In one study, 41% of the men achieved successful intercourse in 50% or more attempts with 3 mg of apomorphine SL, compared with 33% of men who took a 2-mg dose. In fact, apomorphine SL continued to produce a higher number of successful erections than placebo, regardless of whether the erectile dysfunction was mild, moderate, or severe. As would be expected, the success rate with apomorphine was better for those men with milder forms of erectile dysfunction, ranging from 28% in men with severe erectile dysfunction to 68% in men with mild erectile dysfunction. Apomorphine SL was also found to be more effective than placebo in patients whose erectile dysfunction was caused by coronary artery disease (40%), benign prostatic hyperplasia (53%), hypertension (44%), and diabetes mellitus (38%). Long-term studies at 12 and 18 months after the beginning of therapy demonstrated that if the medication was effective, that effectiveness persisted for at least 18 months after therapy was initiated.

Patient and partner assessment of the efficacy of apomorphine using the IIEF and the BSFI demonstrated an improvement in all IIEF domains except for sexual desire. The improvements in scores for erectile function, intercourse satisfaction, overall satisfaction, and orgasmic function were at least twice as high in the group that used apomorphine SL than in the placebo group, with sexual desire being the only parameter that remained unchanged.

The restoration of sexual ability with apomorphine SL is quick, usually occurring within 18–19 minutes after taking the medication. Some men note a response as soon as 10 minutes after taking the medication.

In clinical studies of apomorphine SL, side effects—when they occurred—were typically transient and mild. No treatment-related deaths or drug-related serious adverse effects were reported. The most common adverse events were nausea and yawning (3.9% and 4.6%, respectively). Dizziness and **somnolence**

Somnolence
Sleepiness, unnatural drowsiness.

143

(sleepiness) were also reported (4.0% and 2.8%, respectively). There appeared to be a dose-dependent incidence of adverse events, with the frequency of adverse events being higher when patients took the 3-mg dose. When nausea was experienced, it was felt to be mild in 68% and moderate in 32% of men taking either the 2- or the 3-mg dose. Most men in the studies did not take antiemetics, and very few (0.7%) dropped out because of the nausea. The incidence of nausea appeared to be decreased at the 3-mg dose if the patient started at the 2-mg dose first and increased to 3 mg subsequently.

Vasovagal attack

A transient vascular and neurogenic reaction marked by pallor (white, ghost-like look), sweating, slow heart rate, and lowering of the blood pressure.

The most clinically significant adverse event that occurred with apomorphine SL use was a transient **vasovagal attack,** which consisted of a sudden, transient loss of consciousness with spontaneous full recovery. This complication occurred in fewer than 0.2% of patients who participated in clinical trials of apomorphine SL, and its incidence appeared to be lower if the patients first started at the 2-mg dose and took it a few times before increasing to the 3-mg dose if the 2-mg dose was not satisfactory. Most patients who experienced a syncopal episode experienced certain symptoms before this episode— namely, moderate or severe nausea, dizziness, vomiting, pallor, flushing, hot flashes, and/or sweating. Men who experienced one syncopal episode did not experience another syncopal episode with subsequent use of apomorphine.

82. How might apomorphine compare with sildenafil (Viagra)?

Apomorphine is not approved for use in the United States, and to date no studies have been performed in the United States that compared this medication with sildenafil. Because prior studies of both medications may not have been performed or analyzed in the same way, it is difficult to compare their results. Future studies may provide more information that is relevant to this question.

83. What is yohimbine?

Yohimbine is an oral medication that acts primarily in the brain (centrally). How it exerts an effect on erectile function is not well understood, and study results are conflicting in regard to its effectiveness. Currently, because not enough information is available to demonstrate a clear-cut superiority of yohimbine over placebo, this medication is not recommended as a first-line therapy for erectile dysfunction. Side effects of yohimbine occur in 10–30% of individuals; they are usually mild and include agitation, anxiety, headache, mild increase in blood pressure, increased urinary output, and upset stomach.

Yohimbine is not recommended as a first-line therapy for erectile dysfunction.

84. What are the therapies currently under investigation for erectile dysfunction? How can I try one?

Investigational therapies are not approved by the FDA for the treatment of erectile dysfunction, so you will not be able to purchase them at your local pharmacy. In fact, the only way that you will be able to try one of these therapies is to participate in a clinical trial. To find out whether any clinical trials are happening in your area, you can contact your local urologist's office or, if there is an academic teaching hospital near you, contact the urologist's office there. Be aware that these clinical trials are often random-ized, **double-blind,** placebo-controlled studies. In other words, if you enroll in the study, there is no guarantee that you will get the study medication (i.e., you may get the placebo); the decision of whether you do get the study medication will be made randomly (randomized); and neither you nor the physician will know for sure which medication you are taking (double-blind). Before your enroll-ment, the physician running the study will review the study design with you and will discuss the likeli-hood that you will actually receive the medication.

Oral Therapies

PDE-5 Inhibitors

Two phosphodiesterase type 5 (PDE-5) inhibitors are currently under investigation for erectile dysfunction. SLx-2101 (SurfaceLogix) is a PDE-5 inhibitor with a relatively long half-life of as much as 48 hours. Avanafil (Vivus) appears to have a more rapid onset of action and a shorter half-life than SLx-2101.

L-Arginine

L-Arginine is a precursor of nitric oxide (i.e., nitric oxide is formed from L-arginine), and it is hoped that increasing the amount of L-arginine available will increase the level of nitric oxide. Recall that nitric oxide stimulates the production of cGMP, which in turn tells the cavernosal smooth muscle and the cavernosal arter-ies to relax and dilate, thereby increasing blood flow to the penis and producing an erection (see Questions 4 and 44). To date, only small studies are available regard-ing the use of L-arginine for erectile dysfunction, and these studies have not shown that this drug is superior

Double-blind

Pertaining to a study, a situation in which neither the patient nor the physician is aware of which med-ication the patient is receiving.

to placebo. L-Arginine may cause mild lowering of the blood pressure and fluctuations in heart rate. Nausea, vomiting, diarrhea, headache, flushing, and numbness have also been reported as side effects with L-arginine.

Trazodone

Medications that have been studied as treatments for erectile dysfunction but are not considered first-line therapies include trazodone, an oral psychiatric medication that was found to cause priapism in a small number of men who were taking it for psychiatric problems. In recognition of this effect, trazodone was then studied to see whether it could be used to treat erectile dysfunction. The data regarding the use of trazodone are conflicting, and this agent is not currently recommended as a first-line therapy for erectile dysfunction. Side effects of trazodone include dry mouth and fatigue.

Topical Therapies

Topical alprostadil (Topiglan) is under investigation for erectile dysfunction. This therapy works much like MUSE and injection therapy. It differs in that the man would just apply the gel to the surface of the glans (the tip of the penis), and skin penetration enhancers would then promote absorption of the medication through the penile skin and into the corpora cavernosa. Because it is composed of prostaglandin E_1, topical alprostadil has the same side effects associated with prostaglandin E_1—namely, penile burning and discomfort. In addition, clinical studies found more penile skin irritation in patients who took topical alprostadil than in the group taking a placebo. In a small preliminary study, 69% of men who took this drug achieved an erection sufficient for intercourse, compared with 17% of men who took a placebo.

Injection Therapies

Vasoactive Intestinal Peptide

Vasoactive

Affecting the size (diameter) of blood vessels.

Although **vasoactive** intestinal peptide does appear to play a role in erectile function, the use of this drug alone has not resulted in erections of adequate rigidity to allow vaginal penetration. When vasoactive intestinal peptide is used in tandem with phentolamine, it does appear to produce a significant improvement in erectile function. In one study of 183 men who had not responded to other therapies and who used both vasoactive intestinal peptide and phentolamine, researchers noted an 82% response rate with the combination therapy. An advantage of this combination is that it does not cause penile pain. One third of patients in the study did note transient facial flushing, but priapism occurred in only 0.05%.

Lindisomine

Lindisomine is a nitric oxide donor. Recall that nitric oxide is one of the key mediators in the stimulation of smooth-muscle relaxation and increased blood flow into the penis. Preliminary studies of this drug's efficacy in erectile dysfunction have demonstrated that patients showed a lower response to lindisomine than to prostaglandin therapy. Lindisomine, however, was linked to fewer side effects, such as prolonged erections and priapism. Studies evaluating the efficacy of combination therapy including lindisomine are currently under way.

Forskolin

Forskolin is a plant-based chemical that has been used to increase levels of cAMP in human patients. Recall that cGMP is the main stimulator of cavernosal smooth-muscle relaxation, but that cAMP can also cause cavernosal smooth-muscle relaxation. Studies using forskolin have focused on its use in combination therapy. Preliminary studies have demonstrated that the addition of forskolin to triple P (thus making it a four-drug injection therapy) resulted in a positive response in 61% of men with erectile dysfunction who had not responded to triple P. No adverse effects were noted in this small study.

Surgical Therapies: Interposition Sural Nerve Grafting During Radical Prostatectomy

In recent years, our better understanding of the pelvic anatomy and modifications of surgical techniques have dramatically decreased the morbidity and mortality associated with radical prostatectomy. Nevertheless, despite our growing knowledgebase about the location and function of the pelvic nerves that supply erectile function, and despite modifications in surgical techniques intended to spare these nerves, the incidence of erectile dysfunction after radical prostatectomy remains high, even in bilateral nerve-sparing radical prostatectomy. When both nerves are spared, potency rates are reported to be as high as 71% but are generally closer to the 30–60% range. When both neurovascular bundles are deliberately taken, as is necessary with certain prostate cancers, the incidence of postoperative erectile function is quite low. To date, attempts at better localization of these nerves at the time of surgery using an intraoperative stimulating device, Cavermap Surgical Aid (Uromed), have met with variable success.

Researchers have been investigating the use of **interposition** sural nerve grafting during radical prostatectomy in hopes that it will restore postoperative erectile

Interposition

The act of placing between.

149

function. In interposition nerve grafting, a segment of nerve is removed from one area of the body and placed in another area of the body to replace a damaged nerve. For example, the sural nerve, which is located in the leg, has been used to replace nerves in the arm and the face. The piece of sural nerve serves as a framework for the regeneration of the damaged nerve and promotes growth of new nerve tissue in an orderly manner.

Use of sural nerve grafting for nerve reconstruction in prostate cancer surgery started in the early 1990s but did not really gain momentum until 1997. Since then, several centers throughout the United States, including John's Hopkins University (Baltimore, Maryland) and Baylor College of Medicine (Houston, Texas), have been performing this surgery in carefully selected cases. Because the success of this procedure depends on the regrowth of the damaged nerve and because nerves grow slowly (1 mm/day), it may take as long as 2–3 months for adequate growth of the nerve to occur and as long as 15 months for the "new" nerve tissue to function properly. Thus the maximal results of this procedure may not become apparent until 3 years after the surgery.

A preliminary report on 12 men who underwent bilateral sural nerve grafting and were available for follow-up 1–2 years after the surgery demonstrated that four patients (33%) had spontaneous erections on their own. Five men (41%) had partial erections, and three of these men responded to sildenafil (Viagra). Thus a total of nine men had adequate erectile function with minimal or no additional intervention following this procedure. Side effects of bilateral sural nerve grafting were related to the removal of the sural nerve, such that the patient may have a small area of numbness on the lateral aspect of the foot.

This procedure is still considered investigational and is offered only at a limited number of institutions in the United States. If you are interested in gathering more information about this procedure, a local urologist may be able to direct you to the center closest to you that performs this surgery.

Gene Therapies

Gene therapy—the altering of genes in an attempt to affect their function—is another area in which researchers are seeking treatments for erectile dysfunction. Preliminary studies in animal models have shown that different types of gene therapy may be effective for erectile dysfunction associated with diabetes mellitus and with nerve-related injuries such as those associated with post-radical prostatectomy. At present, this research remains investigational and only preliminary results are available.

Gene therapy

The deliberate alteration of genes in an attempt to affect their function.

85. Can I combine therapies?

To minimize your risk of priapism, you are well advised not to use more than one form of therapy for erectile dysfunction within a 24-hour period. In some cases, when you have not responded to various forms of monotherapy (a single therapy at a time), you might want to discuss the use of combined therapy with your urologist. One of the major limitations of combined therapy is the cost; another drawback is the enhanced potential for side effects.

Studies using a combination of oral sildenafil (Viagra; 100 mg) and intraurethral alprostadil (MUSE; 1000 mg) in men who had not responded to either medication when it was given alone showed that combining the two drugs led to an improvement in erectile function and satisfaction with intercourse in many men. In this study, the men did not start out on the maximum dose of both medications; rather, they gradually increased their dosages until the desired result was achieved.

Oral sildenafil has also been used in combination with intracavernous injection therapy. When sildenafil was used in combination with triple P injection therapy, a higher incidence of dizziness was noted. One concern is that this dizziness may reflect an increase of sildenafil's hypotensive effect by the papaverine in the triple P; for this reason, combination therapy should be used with caution in individuals with cardiovascular disease. Such complications are another reason why combined therapy should be dictated by your urologist, not attempted on your own.

Small studies have been performed to look at the effect of combinations including an alpha blocker as treatments for erectile dysfunction. Alpha blockers block the alpha receptor and cause smooth-muscle relaxation; they are often used as therapies for benign prostatic hyperplasia and high blood pressure. One such medication, doxazosin (Cardura), has been used in combination with either intraurethral alprostadil or intracavernosal injection therapy in men who have not responded to either of the latter therapies used alone. The rationale for using alpha blockers in such cases is that they also cause smooth-muscle relaxation, but via a different mechanism than alprostadil. The combina-

Studies using a combination of oral sildenafil (Viagra; 100 mg) and intraurethral alprostadil (MUSE; 1000 mg) in men who had not responded to either medication when it was given alone showed that combining the two drugs led to an improvement in erectile function and satisfaction with intercourse in many men. In this study, the men did not start out on the maximum dose of both medications; rather, they gradually increased their dosages until the desired result was achieved.

Oral sildenafil has also been used in combination with intracavernous injection therapy. When sildenafil was used in combination with triple P injection therapy, a higher incidence of dizziness was noted. One concern is that this dizziness may reflect an increase of sildenafil's hypotensive effect by the papaverine in the triple P; for this reason, combination therapy should be used with caution in individuals with cardiovascular disease. Such complications are another reason why combined therapy should be dictated by your urologist, not attempted on your own.

Small studies have been performed to look at the effect of combinations including an alpha blocker as treatments for erectile dysfunction. Alpha blockers block the alpha receptor and cause smooth-muscle relaxation; they are often used as therapies for benign prostatic hyperplasia and high blood pressure. One such medication, doxazosin (Cardura), has been used in combination with either intraurethral alprostadil or intracavernosal injection therapy in men who have not responded to either of the latter therapies used alone. The rationale for using alpha blockers in such cases is that they also cause smooth-muscle relaxation, but via a different mechanism than alprostadil. The combina-

Caution is advised when combining therapies, and you should not use more than one therapy for erectile dysfunction without the prior approval of your urologist.

PART FIVE

Talking About and Living With Erectile Dysfunction

How does one bring up the subject of erectile dysfunction?

More ...

86. *How does one bring up the subject of erectile dysfunction?*

Bob's Comment:

In the early 1990s, as I felt a lessened sexual drive and decreased erectile function, I discussed the situation with my endocrinologist, who was treating me for my diabetes. She suggested that I see one of the physicians specializing in urologic problems. My first inclination was to do nothing. This was normal—people my age experience a decrease in their sexual drive and function, I thought. After discussing the situation with my wife, I reluctantly made an appointment to see the urologist.

My appointment date finally arrived. The waiting room at the urology department was quite busy with people of all ages seeking care. I took my place in line, still edgy about proceeding. Any excuse to abort this visit would have sent me to my car in no time! Finally, I was called by the urology nurse, who questioned me matter-of-factly as to my overall health and specifically about my "sexual problem." I cavalierly responded to all questions, as personal as they were. Suddenly, the doctor appeared, accompanied by a urology resident. The doctor was a woman in her 30s, taller than I, who radiated an aura of confidence and efficiency—no nonsense here. Yet I found her to be the type that guys liked to be with. Immediately, I was pleasantly at ease answering her questions and those of her associate. The physical examination of my private area seemed as routine as going through a grocery checkout line. This was clinical. I had the feeling that my situation was no different than hundreds of other men who had preceded me with these same problems. Suddenly, I felt mainstreamed, a willing and active participant in the pursuit of improving my sexuality.

It is often very difficult for a person to bring up the subject of erectile dysfunction, particularly if the topic is not broached by your primary care provider or urologist. Feelings of low self-esteem, guilt, and anxiety can make it difficult to acknowledge that there is a problem. Secondly, the fear of how the doctor will respond can also make one anxious about addressing sexual dysfunction. Everyone fears the casual physician response of "You can't have sex, it will kill you," or "Aren't you too old for sex?" or the insurance company attitude of the ability to participate in sex as being "a pleasure in life and not a medical necessity." Fears of what will occur after one brings up the issue may also prevent one from discussing the topic of erectile dysfunction. Lastly, the worry that "it is all in your mind" may also be a limiting factor. There are several key issues to keep in mind as you are deciding when and how to bring up the discussion of erectile dysfunction:

1. In most men, there is an underlying medical cause of the erectile dysfunction.

2. These medical conditions that cause erectile dysfunction may cause you further harm if not recognized and treated.

3. Even if your erectile troubles are psychological, you can still benefit from treatment, and treatment of your erectile dysfunction along with help dealing with stresses, anxieties, and depression may allow you to have a better quality of life.

4. 50% of men age 40 years and older have some degree of erectile dysfunction, so you are not alone.

5. If your physician does not appear interested in helping you with your erectile dysfunction, find a new one who is interested and willing to help you; they are out there—you just have to be willing to "shop around."

6. If you are open-minded and willing to try various treatment options, you will find something that works for you.

7. Your erectile troubles do not just affect you, they affect your partner, too. Discuss the situation with your partner and work on it as a team—it can help strengthen your relationship. All in all, you cannot lose by bringing the subject up. Do not wait until it dawns on your physician that you have erectile dysfunction; years could pass by. A call to your local hospital or urologist's office can help identify physicians who specialize in erectile dysfunction.

87. What are the psychosocial factors involved in treating erectile dysfunction?

When one partner has troubles with sexual function, both partners are affected. Thus, the more realistic, but sometimes not practical, approach is to work with both partners to restore a healthy physical and emotional outlook for both and to improve their satisfaction with treatments for erectile dysfunction. In order to achieve this goal, it is important that both the patient and the partner are involved in the diagnostic and treatment phases, and that the couple understands the normal erectile process and what may cause problems with erections. It is important to dispel any **myths** (i.e., popular beliefs or traditions that are unfounded or unproven) about erectile dysfunction. It is essential that one understands each partner's reaction to the erectile dysfunction and that person's manner of dealing with the problem. Treatment options need to be discussed clearly, and the benefits, risks, and likelihood of success should be reviewed. Each couple's expectations and relationship are different, and it is important

Myth

A popular belief or tradition that is unfounded and unproven.

that the couple makes a plan for re-establishing their sexual and emotional relationship based on their own physical and emotional responses.

88. I am embarrassed about my erectile troubles and have found myself avoiding my wife/partner. How do I discuss this with my wife/partner?

Bob's Comment:

The question of not discussing erectile dysfunction with your partner is rather moot. This is not a solitary act. It takes two to tango.

Compare this to the situation of a big league relief pitcher being hammered for two home runs for a total of six runs in one inning. How does he avoid discussing this distressing outing to the inquiring reporters, especially if this is his third poor performance in a row? He must discuss it. Like the big leaguer, after a number of subpar sexual performances, you cannot avoid a discussion with your spouse or partner.

I recall when I first started having troubles. After the first poor or marginal sexual effort, I shrugged it off as "I must be a little tired"; after the second, "I guess I am trying too hard"; and then after the third subpar performance, I realized that "something is wrong." I think it is at that time, the realization that things just aren't working properly, that one should discuss things as a couple. Address each individual's needs and desires, and if interested, go forward to find out why this is occurring and what can be done about it. I cannot emphasize enough the need for communication.

It is not uncommon for men with erectile dysfunction to try to avoid sex to avoid having to acknowledge and discuss their erectile troubles. Unfortunately, many men see their lack of erections as a failure, or a lack of manliness, and not what they often truly are, which is a symptom of some underlying medical or psychological disease process. The man may or may not be aware of how common this problem is and may feel that he alone is singled out in this problem. This feeling of failure and lack of manliness often makes men retreat. They avoid discussions with their partner, and they may refrain from simple intimacies, like kissing and hugging, in fear of where it may lead. Unfortunately, what the men often do not realize is that their wife/partner is aware of what is going on, but the wife/partner may feel that they are at fault, that they are no longer sexually attractive to the man, or that their wife/partner is no longer interested in them. These misunderstandings can lead to greater confusion and strains on your relationship. If you discuss this openly in the beginning, both parties can realize that no one is at fault, and no one is to blame. This is a time to reflect and discuss what parts of the sexual intimacy are important to each other, and whether restoration of erectile function is needed by one or both partners for them to participate in a mutually rewarding sexual relationship.

It is not uncommon for men with erectile dysfunction to try to avoid sex to avoid having to acknowledge and discuss their erectile troubles.

89. If I don't have a primary care provider, who should I see to have my erectile dysfunction evaluated and treated?

In this situation, the best thing to do would be to call your local urologist's office to see whether any of the local urologists treat men with erectile dysfunction. Usually, one or more urologists in each practice treats erectile dysfunction. If you do not have a primary care provider and have not seen one in the past, then a more extensive initial evaluation, consisting of more laboratory testing and even a cardiac evaluation, depending on your age and overall health, may be required. If any medical conditions, such as diabetes or high cholesterol level, are detected during this evaluation, you will need to establish a relationship with a primary care provider. Your urologist will be able to assist you with this.

90. I feel stressed and depressed. Is that a common feeling in men with erectile dysfunction?

Bob's Comment:

This is Bob Stanley again, addressing a subject about which I know little. However, I will offer my insights, whatever it is worth.

No longer being able to perform sexually causes anxiety and self-doubt, but don't let it cause undue depression or excessive stress.

When you are unable to perform, there usually are prolonged periods of sexual abstinence. I am certain that this causes the partner to question whether she is still sexually appealing to you. TALK TO HER. This mutual self-doubt should be openly discussed, emphasizing that the problem is a physical one rather than one of lack of desire or caring. In this way, neither partner feels that they are the cause of the problem.

Once you have identified that there is a problem with erectile function, it is incumbent on you and your partner to determine what type of medical help, if any, you are going to proceed with. To let the problem go unresolved indefinitely can certainly lead to feelings of low self-esteem and subsequently to depression and certainly stress.

In these times of developing scientific knowledge and the availability of qualified and experienced physicians dealing with sexual troubles, from both a psychological and a medical point of view, you do yourself a disservice in not at least discussing your problem with your primary care provider and perhaps seeing a specialist.

As Mr. Stanley has indicated, there is no question that erectile dysfunction can have an impact beyond just the sexual aspect. Erectile dysfunction has been associated with low self-esteem, decreased quality of life, depression, and relationship problems.

Many men are not aware of the prevalence of erectile dysfunction and are amazed when they learn that 50% of men over the age of 40 years have some degree of erectile dysfunction. It is reassuring to know that you are not alone, that there are many other men your age and perhaps younger who share your problem. Some men see the onset of erectile dysfunction as a sign that they are "getting old" or "falling apart." Many of us fear getting old, and when problems arise, they make us more anxious. Remember that there are age-related changes in erectile function, but getting older does not cause erectile dysfunction.

When faced with erectile dysfunction, some men will automatically assume that they can no longer participate in sex and can no longer fulfill their partner. In response, they become withdrawn, refrain from intimacy, and may become depressed. It is important to avoid this all-too-frequent response. The fact that you do not get an erection does not mean that you cannot be aroused and climax—an erection is not necessary to achieve a climax. Similarly, there are other ways besides penile-vaginal penetration to satisfy your partner. You and your partner may be pleasantly surprised to find that she is one of the 50% of women who find that they have better orgasms with finger stimulation. It is important to discuss and possibly try these alternatives.

Some men view erectile function as a sign of their manliness and therefore believe that loss of erectile function means that one is no longer a "real man." Well, real men get sick, they develop high blood pressure, diabetes mellitus, heart disease, and other medical conditions that can cause erectile dysfunction. Look at erectile dysfunction not as a personal failure, but as a sign that something is going on that you need to investigate to prevent further health problems.

If I can have one last comment on this subject: "If there is a will, there is a way." If the erectile dysfunction bothers you and you are open-minded, then do not let it get you depressed—talk to your primary care provider or make an appointment with a specialist and have it evaluated and treated. You may not respond to the simpler therapies, like Mr. Stanley, but there is a therapy that will work for you, and there are many therapies currently under investigation. The choice is yours—the treatment is out there if you are interested and willing to try it.

91. How do women respond to male erectile dysfunction?

When a man has a problem with erections, the couple has a sexual problem. Some women whose partners have erectile troubles feel inadequate and may blame themselves for the problem. Some women feel hurt and angry because their partners have withdrawn from them physically and emotionally. Sometimes, a woman raised on myths of men being highly sexual and always ready for sex sees her husband's erections as a marker of his feelings—thus, she interprets the absence of an erection as meaning that he does not care for her or find her attractive. The female partner in a couple with potency problems may need as much or more help than the male.

Often, men will say that they feel that they need to restore their erectile function for their wife, that they will not be able to fulfill their partners sexually without an erection. It is interesting to note that up to 50% of woman find that they are able to be satisfied sexually without participating in vaginal-penetration inter-course. In addition, up to 50% note that they are able to achieve a better orgasm with finger stimulation than vaginal penetration. Therefore, one cannot assume that loss of an erection leads to loss of sexual satisfaction for one's partner. It is important to discuss these sexual preferences with each other.

92. What should I do if my doctor does not seem interested in my erectile troubles?

Bob's Comment:

I was fortunate that when I brought up the discussion of the changes in my sexual function with my diabetes doctor, he quickly indicated that there was an individual in the institution who treated male erectile dysfunction. He responded appropriately to my question and arranged for my visit with Dr. Ellsworth.

I think that a perceived disinterest can be more likely in a situation when one is seeing a physician that is not a urologist. That individual may not be aware of the treatments that are currently available or may not feel comfortable using these therapies. Or that individual may have difficulty discussing the topic of erectile dysfunction or may feel personally that it is not an important issue. If your doctor cannot address your needs, then insist on a referral to a qualified urologist. If your doctor does not do that for you, call your insurance plan and make sure that you can make an appointment with a urologist on your own. It is nice to know that there are urologists today who are interested in treating male erectile and sexual dysfunction.

Studies have looked at why physicians do not screen for (ask about) erectile dysfunction, particularly in high-risk patients. There are several reasons why this may not occur:

- The physician does not want to ask the question because if the patient says "yes," the physician does not know what to do next.
- The physician does not feel comfortable discussing the topic of sexual function.
- The physician is concerned that asking about sexual dysfunction will offend the patient.
- There may be **gender** or generational obstacles that make the physician uncomfortable asking the question.

Gender

The category to which an individual is assigned on the basis of sex, either male or female.

- As physicians, we often feel the need to justify what we do, and unless we can come up with a clear-cut reason why we should ask, we do not.
- The physician may feel that treatment of erectile dysfunction is "not important" and takes up too much time.
- The physician is not aware of the key risk factors for erectile dysfunction.

Thus, the reason for not asking or responding to your suggestions is often not related to you but is often related to "comfort" factors in discussing erectile dysfunction, physician knowledge of the problem, and time constraints. Clearly, as Mr. Stanley indicated, if your physician does not ask, bring it up. If you do not get an adequate response from your doctor, ask to be referred to a specialist. It is your life, and the sooner you start the evaluation, the sooner you can move forward into treatment.

93. Can my partner come to my clinic appointment(s) with me?

It would be wonderful if you could bring your partner to the clinic appointment with you. All too often, in this day and age when both partners are usually working, we only see the man. But erectile dysfunction is a "couples problem," and bringing your partner would help greatly.

During visits, men often note that they are not sure how their partner is going to respond to a certain therapy or state that their partner has concerns about cardiac issues. If the partner is present at the appointment, such issues can be discussed.

With some of the more involved therapies, such as injection therapy, the vacuum device, and the penile prosthesis, it is very helpful to have the partner present during the discussion and demonstration of its use. Some men may find it difficult to inject themselves and may feel more comfortable with their partner performing the injection. Similarly, some men may have difficulty with the pump of the penile prosthesis. Again, it may be easier for the partner to use the pump.

Because erectile dysfunction is a couple's problem, the presence of both partners allows each to address their own concerns. Middle-aged and older female partners may have concerns about their own sexuality and may suffer from problems like atrophic vaginitis. These issues can be addressed if she is present during the visit, and appropriate referrals for her can be made, if necessary.

With some of the more involved therapies, it is very helpful to have the partner present during the discussion and demonstration of its use.

94. Is there a role for sex therapy in the treatment of erectile dysfunction?

Yes, there is often a role for sex therapy in the treatment of erectile dysfunction. You do not have to have psychogenic erectile dysfunction to potentially benefit from sex therapy. Sexual problems do not occur in isolation, nor are their effects limited only to the sexual arena. Sexual problems can be associated with relationship difficulties, decreased self-esteem, anxiety, and depression.

There is often a role for sex therapy in the treatment of erectile dysfunction.

Sex therapy is very effective in helping people understand both the physiologic and the psychological aspects of erectile dysfunction. It also helps people identify and deal with unrealistic expectations and negative self-images, understand their partner's sexual needs and requirements, and dispel any myths about sexuality and sexual function that the patient and his partner may have. It also allows for help with relationship issues, such as intimacy conflicts, power and control struggles, and trust issues, which may be just as important as treatment of the erectile dysfunction in the restoration of a healthy sexual relationship.

Your doctor can help you locate a sex therapist in your area. A sex therapist may be a psychologist or psychiatrist who has a special interest in sexual dysfunction.

95. I have no insurance and I see advertisements in magazines, on the internet, and in flyers that would allow me to buy medications/devices to treat my erectile troubles without having to see a doctor. Wouldn't this be easier and cheaper for me?

This is not the best way to proceed for several reasons:

- Recall that erectile dysfunction is not a disease in and of itself; rather, it is a manifestation of an underlying disease process. Many disease processes or conditions that cause erectile dysfunction can have a significant impact on your health. Thus, the detection of these problems is very important.
- Virtually all medications and therapies have possible side effects and interactions with other medications and therapies. Without the help of a physician to decide whether you are at risk for a drug interaction or a serious side effect from a therapy, you could be at risk for a potentially life-threatening drug inter-

action, such as that resulting from combining Viagra with nitroglycerin-containing products.

- With mail order and on-line companies, you must look into the company. Make sure that you are indeed getting the true medication and not a phony medication, or one with a very similar name that does not work the same way. With vacuum devices, many of the cheaper devices advertised in sex magazines may not have built-in safety protections.

- Often with magazine and on-line ordering, no instructions may be given for the proper use of the medication. Improper use affects the results.

- Some of the advertised medications, particularly herbal and natural medications, have not undergone formal testing whereby the medication is compared with a placebo ("candy pill") to see whether it really works and to identify side effects and risks. Similarly, because it is an herbal or natural medication, do not assume that it is always going to be good for you. Many of these herbal medications can interact with other medications, so again, it is important to involve a physician.

So although it appears tempting, or less involved, or it bypasses the need to discuss a difficult topic, ordering "sex therapies" without seeing a physician and being appropriately evaluated and treated for your erectile troubles is not the ideal way to go. It may cost you more in dollars and in time in the long run, and it could be very dangerous.

Some of the pharmaceutical companies offer financial assistance with some of the therapies for erectile dysfunction. Ask your physician about these programs. If your physician is unaware of this, then ask for the patient information numbers for Pfizer, Pharmacia, Timm, and the other pharmaceutical companies that produce therapies for erectile dysfunction. Pharmacia and Pfizer both provide financial assistance for qualified individuals for the treatment of erectile dysfunction (see Question 100).

96. Sometimes I wake up at night and I have an erection. Does that mean that my erectile troubles are in my head, psychogenic?

No, not necessarily. Nocturnal erections occur via a different mechanism than sexually aroused erections and also serve a different purpose. When you awaken with an erection at night or in the morning, unless you have awakened your partner and have tried to have intercourse, you have no real idea as to whether or not the erection is rigid enough for penetration or would last long enough for completion of sexual performance.

The presence of nocturnal or early morning erections is a good sign. First, it appears that one role of nocturnal erections is to bring increased blood, and therefore increased oxygen, to the penis to keep the tissues healthy. This is important because it may decrease the risk of penile scarring and loss of penile length. Secondly, the presence of nocturnal/early morning erections means that some blood is able to get into the penis, which increases your chances of responding to medical therapy.

So do not be frustrated by the fact that nocturnal or early morning erections occur despite your inability to have an adequate erection when aroused. Rather, look at it as a positive sign that you will most likely have a positive response to medical therapy.

If at times you do not notice any nocturnal erections or early morning erections, do not become too alarmed. The occurrence of nocturnal or early morning erections varies with your quality of sleep. If you are stressed, depressed, or anxious or are have trouble sleeping or nightmares, this may prevent nocturnal erections.

97. Does insurance cover a penile prosthesis?

Bob's Comment:

Since I have diabetes, I was lucky (a fringe benefit for the diabetics of the world)—both Medicare and my private insurance paid for the procedure. Beforehand, I called Medicare and my private insurance company to determine whether implantation of a penile prosthesis would be covered. They both said that since the problem of erectile dysfunction was medically induced (the diabetes), it would be covered as long as my physician submitted a letter outlining the medical necessity. Dr. Ellsworth cheerily complied. Note: It is helpful to use the right language and medical buzz words when calling the age 20-something insurance clerk who one senses can't wait to discuss your call with her workmates after signoff.

It is well worth verifying coverage of the procedure in the beginning, because an implant procedure is very expensive, considering the surgical charges, the operating room charges, the prosthesis itself, and the overnight hospital stay expenses.

As Mr. Stanley indicated, if one has an identifiable medical condition that is causing the erectile dysfunction, most insurance companies pay for the prosthesis, but it is important to verify this early on. Some managed-care companies may restrict the type of prosthesis that they cover. Again, this is something to identify early and settle before the surgery. If your insurance company does not cover placement of a penile prosthesis, then you can talk with the hospital's social service department about other available avenues for assistance or a payment plan.

98. I have angina. Is sex bad for me?

The answer to this question is not a simple yes or no. The response depends on several factors: what your exercise level is, how often you have angina, what medications you are taking, and how severe your heart disease is.

If you are an active individual, that is if you jog, play tennis, or get some form of regular exercise, and do not experience angina routinely with this exercise, then your risk of having angina during intercourse would be lower. If you experience angina with minimal physical exertion, such as walking to the mailbox to pick up your mail, then sex may cause angina for you.

If you have very unstable angina and require sublingual nitroglycerin on a regular basis and have severe heart disease that cannot be corrected, then realistically you have an increased risk of having angina during intercourse.

If you have controlled angina, you may be able to participate in intercourse; however, anyone who requires the use of nitroglycerin will not be able to use the oral therapy Viagra for restoration of his erectile function, because the simultaneous use of

Viagra and nitroglycerin within a 24-hour period can have serious effects, perhaps life-threatening. The two medications, when combined, can lead to significant drops in blood pressure, up to 70 points, which can lead to decreased blood flow to the heart. Some deaths have been reported in men using the two medications within a 24-hour period. Thus, if you have a history of angina and have been prescribed nitroglycerin in the past, it is very important for you and your physician to review your level of physical activity and your likelihood of needing nitroglycerin during intercourse before considering the use of Viagra.

You may still develop angina with intercourse if you use other forms of therapy for erectile dysfunction. The difference is that they will not interfere with the simultaneous use of that therapy and nitroglycerin, and therefore you can go ahead and take a sublingual nitroglycerin.

99. What happens if I have chest pain during intercourse?

As with any other activity that may precipitate chest pain (angina), the first thing that you should do if you have chest pain during intercourse is to stop what you are doing. If you have taken Viagra for your erectile dysfunction, then you cannot take any nitroglycerin-containing medications for a full 24 hours after you took the Viagra. If your chest pain does not resolve with stopping your activity, then you should go to your local emergency room. It is very important for you or your partner to inform the emergency room staff that you have taken Viagra within the previous 24 hours. The emergency room staff will then use different medications to treat your angina that will not interact with the Viagra.

100. Where can I get more information?

The following resources are available to those who want to learn more:

Organizations

American Urological Association
Health Policy Department
1120 North Charles Street
Baltimore, MD 21201
Tel: 410–223–4367

American Foundation for Urologic Disease (AFUD)
1126 North Charles Street
Baltimore, MD 21201
Tel: 800–242–2383
www.afud.org

US TOO International, Inc.
Prostate Cancer Support Groups
930 North York Road, Suite 50
Hinsdale, IL 60521
www.ustoo.com

International Society of Impotence Research
Contact: Mrs. Marianne Mulder
University Hospital Nijmegen, Department of Urology
P.O. Box 9101, 6500 HB Nijmegen
The Netherlands
Tel: +31–24–3613920

The Impotence Association
PO Box 10296
London SW17 9WH
United Kingdom
www.impotence.org.uk

Web Sites

www.urohealth.org, supported by Abbott Laboratories

www.medformation.com, supported by Allina Hospitals &
  Clinics

www.menshealthforum.org.uk, sponsored by the UK Men's
  Health Forum

www.drkoop.com

www.viagra.com, supported by Pfizer Inc.

Books and Publications

The Treatment of Organic Erectile Dysfunction: A Patient's Guide.
The American Urological Association Erectile Dysfunction Clin-
ical Guidelines Panel. Copies can be obtained from the AUA
Health Policy Department at the address listed above.

Caverject User's Guide. Produced by Pharmacia. Contact the
Patient Product Information Center at 1–888–691–6813.

Levine SB. *Sexuality in Mid-Life.* New York: Plenum Press,
1998.

Levine SB. *Sexual Life: A Clinician's Guide (Critical Issues in
Psychiatry).* New York: Plenum Press, 1992.

Rosen RC, Leiblum SR, eds. *Erectile Disorders: Assessment and
Treatment.* New York: Guilford Press, 1992.

Abdomen: The part of the body below the ribs and above the pelvic bone that contains organs such as the intestines, the liver, the kidneys, the stomach, the bladder, and the prostate.

Acquired anorgasmia: An inability to have an orgasm owing to the side effects of medical therapy.

Adenoma: A benign, noncancerous tumor in which the cells form glandular structures.

Alpha blockers: A group of medications that may be used to treat the symptoms of benign prostate enlargement. They include doxazosin (Cardura), terazosin (Hytrin), and tamsulosin (Flowmax).

Alprostadil: Prostaglandin E_1. For the treatment of erectile dysfunction, alprostadil comes in several forms—specifically, a suppository that is placed into the urethra (MUSE) or a liquid form that is delivered by intracavernous injection (Caverject or Edex).

Androderm: A topical form (patch) of testosterone used for testosterone replacement therapy.

Androgel: A gel form of testosterone replacement therapy.

Androgens: Hormones that are necessary for the development and function of the male sexual organs and male sexual characteristics (e.g., hair, voice change).

Anejaculation: An inability to ejaculate.

Anesthesia: The loss of feeling or sensation. With respect to surgery, it means the loss of sensation of pain, as it is induced to allow surgery or other painful procedures to be performed. *General anesthesia* is a state of unconsciousness, produced by anesthetic agents, that is marked by the absence of pain sensation over the entire body and a greater or lesser degree of muscle relaxation. *Local anesthesia* is confined to one part of the body. *Spinal anesthesia* is produced by injection of a local anesthetic into the subarachnoid space around the spinal cord.

Aneurysm: Pertaining to a penile prosthesis, an abnormal dilation of the prosthesis related to weakening of a part of the cylinder.

Angina: Pain in the chest, with a feeling of suffocation, that occurs with decreased blood flow and oxygenation to the heart.

Anorexia: Loss of appetite.

Anorgasmia: Failure to experience an orgasm during sex. See also *Acquired anorgasmia* and *Congenital anorgasmia*.

Antidepressant: Medication prescribed to relieve depression.

Arteriography: A test for identifying and locating arterial disease in the penis, using ultrasound and injected contrast to find constricted or blocked arteries.

Artery: A blood vessel that carries oxygenated blood from the heart to other parts of the body.

Atherosclerosis: Hardening of the arteries, often related to smoking.

Autoinflation: Pertaining to a penile prosthesis, the spontaneous inflation of the prosthesis without manual pumping.

Axial rigidity: The rigidity as measured along the axis or length of the penis.

Benign: A growth that is noncancerous.

Benign prostatic hyperplasia (BPH): Noncancerous enlargement of the prostate.

Bilateral: Affecting both sides.

Biopsy: The removal of small sample(s) of tissue for examination under the microscope.

Butterfly needle: A small needle that has tubing attached to it.

Catheter: A hollow tube that allows for fluid drainage from or injection into an area.

Caverject: A form of injection therapy produced by Pfizer. It contains prostaglandin E_1.

Cavernosography: A technique used to visualize areas of venous leak. It involves the injection of a cavernous smooth-muscle dilator (e.g., prostaglandin E_1 or trimix), followed by placement of a butterfly needle into the corpora, instillation of a contrast agent into the corpora, and x-ray photographs to visualize the sites of venous leak.

Cavernosometry: A somewhat invasive technique used to determine whether a venous leak is present.

Central nervous system: The portion of the nervous system consisting of the brain and the spinal cord.

cGMP: A neurotransmitter that causes relaxation of the arteries and smooth muscles in the penis to permit increased blood flow into the penis.

Cholesterol: A fat-like substance that is important to certain body functions but that, when present in excessive amounts, contributes to unhealthy fatty deposits in the arteries that may interfere with blood flow.

Cialis: See *Tadalafil.*

Complication: An undesirable result of a treatment, surgery, or medication.

Congenital anorgasmia: A rare form of anorgasmia that is thought to be a product of an overly strict or repressive attitude toward sex.

Congestive heart failure: An inability of the heart to pump blood adequately, leading to swelling and fluid in the lungs.

Corona: The area of the penis just before the glans.

Corpora cavernosa: The two cylindrical structures in the penis that are composed of the penile erectile tissue. They are located on the top of the penis (singular: corpus cavernosum).

Corpus spongiosum: One of the three cylindrical structures in the penis. The urethra passes through the corpus spongiosum. It is not involved in erections.

Delayed ejaculation: Taking a longer time to ejaculate. This effect is seen with some antidepressants.

Depression: A mental state of depressed mood characterized by feelings of sadness, despair, and discouragement.

Detumescence: Subsidence of swelling or turgor; with respect to erections, loss of rigidity.

Diabetes mellitus: A chronic disease associated with high levels of sugar (glucose) in the blood.

Diagnosis: The identification of the cause or presence of a medical problem or disease.

Digital rectal examination (DRE): The examination of the prostate by placing a gloved finger into the rectum.

Disease: Any change from or interruption of the normal structure or function of any part, organ, or system of the body that presents with characteristic symptoms and signs, and whose cause and prognosis may be known or unknown.

Doppler ultrasonography: Use of a Doppler probe during ultrasound to look at flow through vessels.

Double-blind: Pertaining to a study, a situation in which neither the patient nor the physician is aware of which medication the patient is receiving.

Edex: Alprostadil alfadex. A form of injection therapy produced by Schwarz Pharma. It contains prostaglandin E_1 and works via the same mechanism as Caverject.

Efficacy: The power or ability to produce an effect.

Ejaculation: The release of semen through the penis during orgasm.

Ejaculatory duct: The structure through which the ejaculate passes into the urethra.

Ejaculatory dysfunction: An abnormality of ejaculatory function, such as retrograde ejaculation, premature ejaculation, delayed ejaculation, or anejaculation.

Electroejaculation: Use of an electrical stimulus to induce ejaculation.

Embolization: The introduction of a substance into a blood vessel in an attempt to obstruct (occlude) it.

Emission: A discharge, either voluntary or involuntary, of semen from the ejaculatory duct into the urethra.

Enzyme: A chemical that is produced by living cells that causes chemical reactions to occur while not being changed itself.

Erectile dysfunction: The inability to achieve and/or maintain an erection satisfactory for the completion of sexual performance.

Erection: The process whereby the penis becomes rigid.

Erosion: Destruction of a tissue surface—for example a penile prosthesis eroding through the skin.

Experimental: An untested or unproven treatment or approach to treatment.

External-beam radiation therapy (EBRT): A radiation technique that is used to treat many types of cancer. Beams of high-energy radiation pass through the skin, with the maximal energy being focused on the target organ (e.g., the prostate).

Foley catheter: A catheter that is placed into the bladder via the urethra to drain urine.

Food and Drug Administration (FDA): The federal agency responsible for the approval of prescription medications in the United States.

GAQ: See *Global assessment questionnaire.*

Gender: The category to which an individual is assigned on the basis of sex, either male or female.

Gene therapy: The deliberate alteration of genes in an attempt to affect their function.

Genitalia: The external sexual organs—in the male, the penis, testes, epididymis, and vas deferens.

Genitourinary tract: The urinary system (kidneys, ureters and bladder, and urethra) and the genitalia (in the male, the prostate, seminal vesicles, vas deferens, and testicles).

Glans: The tip of the penis.

Global assessment questionnaire (GAQ): A self-administered questionnaire that allows patients to rate improvement in erectile function.

Glycosylated end-products: A chemical associated with diabetes that may contribute to erectile dysfunction by decreasing nitric oxide activity.

Glycosylated hemoglobin: A chemical in the blood that allows monitoring of blood sugar control in individuals with diabetes mellitus. An elevated $HgbA_{1c}$ is indicative of poor blood sugar control.

Groin: The area between the lower abdomen and the thigh.

Gynecomastia: Enlargement or tenderness of the male breast(s).

Hardening of the arteries: Descriptive expression that commonly refers to a group of diseases (forms of arteriosclerosis) characterized by abnormal thickening and hardening (sclerosis) of arterial walls, in which the arteries lose their elasticity. If the thickening/hardening is significant, it may interfere with blood flow.

Hematoma: A blister-like collection of blood under the skin.

High-density lipoprotein (HDL): "Good" cholesterol.

High-flow priapism: Priapism that occurs secondary to increased arterial flow.

History: An oral or written interview that consists of questions about your medical, social, and sexual background.

Hypercholesterolemia: An excess of cholesterol in the blood.

Hyperprolactinemia: A condition characterized by excess prolactin production. It may be related to a tumor of the pituitary gland but also may be caused by certain medications.

Hypertension: High blood pressure.

Hypogonadism: A condition in which the testes are not producing adequate testosterone. It may occur because of a testicular problem or because of a lack of stimulation of the testes by the brain.

Hypotension: Low blood pressure.

Iatrogenic: Resulting from treatment by a physician, such as from medications, procedures, or surgery.

Impotence: See *Erectile dysfunction.*

Incidence: The rate at which a certain event occurs—for example, the number of new cases of a specific disease that occur during a certain period.

Indication: The reason for doing something.

Inpatient: A patient who is admitted to the hospital for treatment.

Insulin-dependent diabetes mellitus: Diabetes in which the body does not produce sufficient insulin.

Interposition: The act of placing between.

Intracavernous: Into the corpora cavernosa.

Intracavernous pressure: The pressure within the corpora cavernosa, as measured during cavernosography.

Intramuscular (IM): Pertaining to the muscles; injection into the muscle.

Intraurethral: Placed into the urethra.

Intraurethral alprostadil: See *MUSE.*

Investigational: See *Experimental.*

Ischemia: A deficiency of blood flow to an area that compromises the health of the tissue.

Leukemia: A cancer of the blood-forming organs that affects the blood cells.

Levitra: See *Vardenafil.*

Libido: Sexual desire; one's interest in sex.

Local anesthesia: Anesthesia confined to one part of the body.

Low-flow priapism: Priapism that occurs secondary to venous outflow obstruction.

Luteinizing hormone (LH): A chemical produced by the brain that stimulates the testes to produce testosterone.

Migration: Spontaneous change of place.

Morbidity: Diseased condition or state.

Mortality: Death in a population at risk.

MUSE: Intraurethral alprostadil; a small suppository that comes preloaded in a small applicator that is placed into the tip of the penis. The small button at the other end of the suppository is squeezed to release the suppository into the urethra. Gentle rubbing of the penis causes the suppository to dissolve. The prostaglandin is then absorbed through the urethral mucosa and passes into the corpora cavernosa, where it stimulates blood flow into the penis through the cAMP pathway.

Myth: A popular belief or tradition that is unfounded and unproven.

NAION: See *Nonarteritic ischemic optic neuropathy.*

Nerve: A cordlike structure composed of a collection of nerve fibers that conveys impulses between a part of the central nervous system and some other region of the body.

Neurologic: Pertaining to the brain or nerves.

Neurotransmitter: A chemical released from a nerve cell that transmits an impulse to another nerve, cell, or organ.

Nitrate: A form of nitric acid that causes dilation (opening up) of the blood vessels to the heart. Nitroglycerin is a form of nitrate.

Nitric oxide: A chemical in the body that stimulates production of cGMP, which is necessary for erectile function.

Nitroglycerin: A medication that is usually taken sublingually (under the tongue) for the relief of angina. It may also be applied to the chest in a paste form for the prevention of angina.

Nocturnal: Occurring or active at night.

Nocturnal penile tumescence (NPT) study: A specialized study that evaluates the frequency and the quality of nocturnal erections.

Nonarteritic ischemic optic neuropathy (NAION): A sudden, painless loss of vision in one or both eyes. The cause is reduced blood flow to the optic nerve.

Non–insulin-dependent diabetes mellitus: Diabetes in which the body does not respond adequately to insulin.

Noninvasive: Not requiring any incision or insertion of an instrument or substance into the body.

Objective: Perceptible to the external senses; something the physician uses to quantify, measure, or identify.

Occlusion: Blockage of flow.

Occult: Not detectable on gross examination.

Oral: Taken by mouth.

Orchiectomy: Removal of the testicle(s).

Organ: Tissues in the body that work together to perform a specific function (e.g., heart, bladder, penis).

Orgasm: Sexual climax; the culmination of sexual excitement.

Orgasmic dysfunction: Alterations in orgasmic function or the inability to achieve an orgasm.

Orthostatic hypotension: The acute lowering of blood pressure when a person changes from a sitting or lying position to an upright position (standing). Also called postural hypotension.

Palpation: Feeling with the hand or fingers, by applying light pressure.

Parenteral: Administered not by mouth but rather by injection by some other route (e.g., intramuscular, subcutaneous).

PDE-5 inhibitor: See *Phosphodiesterase type 5 inhibitor.*

Pelvis: The part of the body that is framed by the hip bones.

Penile arterial bypass surgery: A surgical procedure that provides an alternative pathway to bring blood flow into the penis and avoids the obstructed artery.

Penile prosthesis: A device that is surgically placed into the penis that allows a man with erectile dysfunction to have an erection.

Penis: The male organ that is used for urination and intercourse.

Perineum: The area under the scrotum.

Peyronie's disease: A benign (noncancerous) condition of the penis that tends to affect middle-aged men. It is characterized by the formation of plaques in the tunica albuginea of the penis and may cause erectile dysfunction.

Phosphodiesterase type 5 (PDE-5): An enzyme that is responsible for the breakdown of cGMP. Inhibition of PDE-5 leads to a buildup of cGMP.

Phosphodiesterase type 5 (PDE-5) inhibitor: A chemical that prevents the function of PDE-5. The use of such an inhibitor leads to an increase in cGMP.

Physiologic: Functioning in a normal range for human physiology.

Pituitary adenoma: A benign tumor of the pituitary gland. An adenoma of the anterior pituitary may produce excessive amounts of prolactin.

Pituitary gland: A gland in the brain that is composed of two parts (lobes), the anterior gland and the posterior gland. The anterior pituitary gland produces a variety of hormones, including luteinizing hormone and prolactin.

Placebo: A fake medication ("sugar pill") or treatment that has no effect on the body and that is often used in experimental studies to determine whether the experimental medication/treatment has an effect.

Polycythemia: An increase in the total red blood cell mass in the blood.

Premature ejaculation: Quick ejaculation. The fourth edition of the

American Psychiatric Association's *Diagnostic and Statistical Manual* outlines three criteria for premature ejaculation: (1) persistent or repeated ejaculation occurs with slight stimulation before, on, or shortly after penetration and before the person wishes it; (2) the disturbance causes considerable anguish or interpersonal difficulty; and (3) the premature ejaculation is not due exclusively to the direct effects of a chemical.

Prevalence: The number of cases of a disease that are present in a population at one given point in time.

Priapism: The persistence of an erection, unassociated with sexual pleasure, that lasts for 6 or more hours. If left untreated, it can lead to penile ischemia and subsequent erectile dysfunction.

Prolactin: One of the hormones produced by the pituitary gland. In males, elevated prolactin levels can lower testosterone levels, decrease libido, and affect erectile function.

Prolonged erection: An erection that lasts longer than 4 hours but less than 6 hours. It may be associated with the use of pharmacologic therapy for erectile dysfunction.

Prostaglandin E_1: A type of prostaglandin that increases the cAMP level, which causes smooth-muscle relaxation.

Prostate: A gland that surrounds the urethra and is located just under the bladder. It produces fluid that is part of the ejaculate (semen). This fluid provides some nutrient to the sperm.

Prosthesis: An artificial device used to replace the lost normal function of a structure or organ in the body.

Psychogenic: Stemming from the mind or psyche.

Quality of life: An evaluation of healthy status relative to the patient's age, expectations, and physical and mental capabilities.

Radial rigidity: Rigidity across the width or radius of the penis.

Radiation therapy: Administration of radiation to treat a disease.

Radical prostatectomy: A surgical procedure for prostate cancer in which the entire prostate and seminal vesicles, and part of the vas deferens, are removed.

Randomized: The process of assigning patients to different forms of treatment in a research study in a random manner.

Rapid eye movement (REM): A phase in the sleep cycle. Nocturnal erections occur during this phase of sleep.

Red blood cells: The cells in the blood that carry oxygen to the tissues.

Resistance: Opposition to blood flow out of the penis.

Retrograde ejaculation: A condition whereby the ejaculate passes backward into the bladder instead of forward out the tip of the penis. This problem frequently occurs after transurethral prostatectomy.

Retroperitoneal lymph node dissection: A procedure to remove lymph nodes adjacent to the site of testicular or prostate cancer.

Risk: The chance or probability that a particular event will or will not happen.

Salvage: A procedure intended to "rescue" a patient who has failed to respond to a prior therapy.

Scrotum: The pouch of skin that contains the testicles.

Selective serotonin reuptake inhibitor (SSRI): A type of medication that is used for depression and for premature ejaculation. Commonly used SSRIs include sertraline, paroxetine, and fluoxetine.

Semen: The thick whitish fluid, produced by glands of the male reproductive system, that carries the sperm (reproductive cells) through the penis during ejaculation.

Sex hormones: Substances (estrogens and androgens) responsible for secondary sex characteristics (e.g., hair growth and voice change in males).

Sexual dysfunction: An abnormality in the function of any component of the sexual response cycle.

Sexual response cycle: The cycle of interest, arousal, climax, ejaculation, and detumescence.

Sickle cell disease/sickle cell trait: A genetically inherited condition in which red blood cells take on an abnormal shape (sickle) in response to decreased oxygenation, dehydration, and acidosis. This abnormal shape makes it difficult for the red blood cells to pass through the blood vessels and leads to blockages of the vessels, causing pain and ischemia to tissues. In the penis, it may lead to priapism. African Americans are especially prone to the sickle cell trait.

Side effect: An undesirable reaction to a medication or treatment.

Sign: Objective evidence of a disease or condition; something that the doctor identifies.

Sildenafil (Viagra): The first effective, FDA-approved oral therapy for erectile dysfunction. Sildenafil is a phosphodiesterase type 5 inhibitor.

Sinusoid: A blood-filled cavernous space. In the penis, these spaces are separated by a network of connective tissues containing muscle cells, small arteries, veins, and nerves.

Somnolence: Sleepiness, unnatural drowsiness.

SSRI: See *Selective serotonin reuptake inhibitor.*

Striant: A transbuccal form of testosterone replacement therapy.

Subjective: Pertaining to or perceived by the affected individual, but not perceptible to the other senses of another person.

Supraphysiologic: Higher than the normal functional state or level in the body.

Symptom: Subjective evidence of a disease; something the patient describes, such as pain in abdomen.

Syncope: A temporary loss of consciousness.

Tachyphylaxis: Decreased response of a patient to a drug that was previously effective.

Tadalafil (Cialis): An oral therapy for erectile dysfunction; a phosphodiesterase type 5 inhibitor with a long half-life (17–21 hours).

Testes: Two male reproductive organs that are located within the scrotum and produce testosterone and sperm. (singular: testis)

Testim: A gel form of testosterone replacement therapy.

Testoderm: A topical form (patch) of testosterone used for testosterone replacement therapy.

Testosterone: The male hormone. It is responsible for secondary sex characteristics, such as hair growth and voice change. Testosterone is also the key hormone involved in sexual desire (libido).

Tissue: A specific type of material in the body (e.g., muscle, hair).

Transdermal: Entering through the skin, as in administration of a drug applied to the skin in an ointment, gel, or patch form.

Transrectal: Through the rectum.

Transrectal ultrasound: Visualization of the prostate by the use of an ultrasound probe placed into the rectum.

Transurethral prostatectomy (TURP): A surgical technique performed under anesthesia in which the surgeon uses a specialized instrument to remove prostatic tissue that is bulging into the urethra and blocking the flow of urine through the urethra. After a TURP, a rim of prostatic tissue remains.

Trazodone: A psychiatric medication that has been reported to cause priapism. Studies using trazodone for the treatment of erectile dysfunction have produced conflicting results. Currently, trazodone is not believed to be a reliable therapy for the treatment of erectile dysfunction.

Tumescence: Condition of being tumid or swollen; with respect to erections, penile rigidity.

Tunica albuginea: The dense, fibrous, elastic sheath enclosing the corpora cavernosa in the penis. Compression of small veins against the tunica albuginea during erection holds back the outflow of blood from the corpora, causing the penis to be rigid.

Ultrasound: A technique used to look at internal organs by measuring reflected sound waves.

Urethra: The tube that a person urinates through.

Urologist: A doctor who specializes in the evaluation and treatment of diseases of the genitourinary tract in men and women.

Vacuum device: A device that is used to provide an erection. It consists of three parts: a cylinder, a pump, and a constricting band. The band is preloaded on the bottom of the cylinder, and the cylinder is placed over the penis. The pump, which is connected to the cylinder, creates a suction that pulls blood into the penis. Because the constricting band is placed at the base of the penis, the blood remains in the penis until the band is removed.

Vardenafil (Levitra): An oral form of erectile dysfunction therapy; a phosphodiesterase type 5 inhibitor.

Vascular: Pertaining to blood vessels.

Vas deferens: The duct that sperm travel through from the testis to the urethra.

Vasoactive: Affecting the size (diameter) of blood vessels.

Vasospasm: Constriction of the arteries.

Vasovagal attack: A transient vascular and neurogenic reaction marked by pallor (white, ghost-like look), sweating, slow heart rate, and lowering of the blood pressure.

Vein: A blood vessel in the body that carries deoxygenated blood from the tissues back to the heart.

Venous leak: The situation in which veins do not compress to prevent blood from draining out of the corpora during erection. Venous leak may also refer to the rare occasions in which abnormally located veins allow for persistent drainage of blood during an erection.

Venous ligation surgery: A surgical procedure in which leaky veins in the penis are ligated to prevent blood from continually flowing out of the penis during erection.

Viagra: See *Sildenafil.*

X-ray: A type of high-energy radiation that can be used at low levels to make images of the internal structure of the body and at high levels for radiation therapy.

Yohimbine: An oral medication that acts primarily in the brain. It has been reported to improve erectile function; however, study results are conflicting, and yohimbine is not recommended as a first-line therapy for erectile dysfunction.

International Index of Erectile Function (IIEF)

A Multidimensional Scale for Assessment of Erectile Dysfunction

These questions ask about the effects your erection problems have had on your sex life **over the past 4 weeks.** Please answer the following questions as honestly and clearly as possible. In answering these questions, the following definitions apply:

- **sexual activity** includes intercourse, caressing, foreplay, and masturbation
- **sexual intercourse** is defined as vaginal penetration of the partner (you entered your partner)
- **sexual stimulation** includes situations like foreplay with a partner, looking at erotic pictures, etc.
- **ejaculate** is the ejection of semen from the penis (or the feeling of this)

1. **Over the past 4 weeks,** how often were you able to get an erection during sexual activity? *Please check one box only.*
   - ❑ No sexual activity
   - ❑ Almost always/always
   - ❑ Most times (much more than half the time)
   - ❑ Sometimes (about half the time)
   - ❑ A few times (much less than half the time)
   - ❑ Almost never/never

2. **Over the past 4 weeks,** when you had erections with sexual stimula-

tion, how often were your erections hard enough for penetration? *Please check one box only.*
   - ❑ No sexual activity
   - ❑ Almost always/always
   - ❑ Most times (much more than half the time)
   - ❑ Sometimes (about half the time)
   - ❑ A few times (much less than half the time)
   - ❑ Almost never/never

The next three questions will ask about the erections you may have had during sexual intercourse.

3. **Over the past 4 weeks,** when you attempted sexual intercourse, how often were you able to penetrate (enter) your partner? *Please check one box only.*
   - ❑ Did not attempt intercourse
   - ❑ Almost always/always
   - ❑ Most times (much more than half the time)
   - ❑ Sometimes (about half the time)
   - ❑ A few times (much less than half the time)
   - ❑ Almost never/never

4. **Over the past 4 weeks,** during sexual intercourse, how often were you able to maintain your erection after you had penetrated (entered) your partner? *Please check one box only.*
   - ❑ Did not attempt intercourse
   - ❑ Almost always/always

❏ Most times (much more than half the time)

❏ Sometimes (about half the time)

❏ A few times (much less than half the time)

❏ Almost never/never

5. **Over the past 4 weeks,** during sexual intercourse, how difficult was it to maintain your erection to completion of intercourse? *Please check one box only.*

❏ Did not attempt intercourse

❏ Extremely difficult

❏ Very difficult

❏ Difficult

❏ Slightly difficult

❏ Not difficult

6. **Over the past 4 weeks,** how many times have you attempted sexual intercourse? *Please check one box only.*

❏ No attempts

❏ 1–2 attempts

❏ 3–4 attempts

❏ 5–6 attempts

❏ 7–10 attempts

❏ 11+ attempts

7. **Over the past 4 weeks,** when you attempted sexual intercourse, how often was it satisfactory for you? *Please check one box only.*

❏ Did not attempt intercourse

❏ Almost always/always

❏ Most times (much more than half the time)

❏ Sometimes (about half the time)

❏ A few times (much less than half the time)

❏ Almost never/never

8. **Over the past 4 weeks,** how much have you enjoyed sexual intercourse? *Please check one box only.*

❏ No intercourse

❏ Very highly enjoyable

❏ Highly enjoyable

❏ Fairly enjoyable

❏ Not very enjoyable

❏ No enjoyment

9. **Over the past 4 weeks,** when you had sexual stimulation or intercourse, how often did you ejaculate? *Please check one box only.*

❏ No sexual stimulation/intercourse

❏ Almost always/always

❏ Most times (much more than half the time)

❏ Sometimes (about half the time)

❏ A few times (much less than half the time)

❏ Almost never/never

10. **Over the past 4 weeks,** when you had sexual stimulation or intercourse, how often did you have the feeling of orgasm (with or without ejaculation)? *Please check one box only.*

❏ No sexual stimulation/intercourse

❑ Almost always/always

❑ Most times (much more than half the time)

❑ Sometimes (about half the time)

❑ A few times (much less than half the time)

❑ Almost never/never

The next two questions ask about sexual desire. Let's define sexual desire as a feeling that may include wanting to have a sexual experience (e.g., masturbation or intercourse), thinking about having sex, or feeling frustrated due to lack of sex.

11. **Over the past 4 weeks,** how often have you felt **sexual desire?** *Please check one box only.*

❑ Almost always/always

❑ Most times (much more than half the time)

❑ Sometimes (about half the time)

❑ A few times (much less than half the time)

❑ Almost never/never

12. **Over the past four weeks,** how would you rate your level of sexual desire? *Please check one box only.*

❑ Very high

❑ High

❑ Moderate

❑ Low

❑ Very low or none at all

13. **Over the past 4 weeks,** how satisfied have you been with your overall sex life? *Please check one box only.*

❑ Very satisfied

❑ Moderately satisfied

❑ About equally satisfied and dissatisfied

❑ Moderately dissatisfied

❑ Very dissatisfied

14. **Over the past 4 weeks,** how satisfied have you been with your sexual relationship with your partner? *Please check one box only.*

❑ Very satisfied

❑ Moderately satisfied

❑ About equally satisfied and dissatisfied

❑ Moderately dissatisfied

❑ Very dissatisfied

15. **Over the past 4 weeks,** how do you rate your confidence that you can get and keep your erection? *Please check one box only.*

❑ Very high

❑ High

❑ Moderate

❑ Low

❑ Very low or none at all

PATIENT INSTRUCTIONS

Sexual health is an important part of an individual's overall physical and emotional well-being. Erectile dysfunction, also known as impotence, is one type of very common medical condition affecting sexual health. Fortunately, there are many different treatment options for erectile dysfunction. This questionnaire is designed to help you and your doctor identify if you may be experiencing erectile dysfunction. If you are, you may choose to discuss treatment options with your doctor.

Each question has several possible responses. Circle the number of the response that best describes your own situation. Please be sure that you select one and only one response for each question.

OVER THE PAST 6 MONTHS:

1. How do you rate your <u>confidence</u> that you could get and keep an erection?

Very low	Low	Moderate	High	Very high
1	2	3	4	5

2. When you had erections with sexual stimulation, <u>how often</u> were your erections hard enough for penetration (entering your partner)?

No sexual activity	Almost never or never	A few times (much less than half the time)	Sometimes (about half the time)	Most times (much more than half the time)	Almost always or always
0	1	2	3	4	5

3. During sexual intercourse, <u>how often</u> were you able to maintain your erections after you had penetrated (entered) your partner?

Did not attempt intercourse	Almost never or never	A few times (much less than half the time)	Sometimes (about half the time)	Most times (much more than half the time)	Almost always or always
0	1	2	3	4	5

4. During sexual intercourse, <u>how difficult</u> was it to maintain your erections after you had penetrated (entered) your partner?

Did not attempt intercourse	Extremely difficult	Very difficult	Difficult	Slightly difficult	Not difficult
0	1	2	3	4	5

5. When you attempted sexual intercourse, <u>how often</u> was it satisfactory for you?

Did not attempt intercourse	Almost never or never	A few times (much less than half the time)	Sometimes (about half the time)	Most times (much more than half the time)	Almost always or always
0	1	2	3	4	5

SCORE_____

Add the numbers corresponding to questions 1–5. If your score is 21 or less, you may want to speak with your doctor.

Index

Page numbers followed by *t* or *f* indicate tables or figures, respectively.

Abdomen, 37, 177
ACTIS venous constrictor, 98
Adenoma
  definition of, 9, 177
  pituitary, 9, 30–31, 183
Aging, 20–21
Alcohol, 27*t*
Alcohol use, 16, 20
Alpha blockers
  combination treatments with, 152–153
  definition of, 83, 177
  and PDE-5 inhibitors, 83–84, 92
Alprazolam (Xanax), 19
Alprostadil
  cavernosometry with, 48–49
  combined with prazosin, 153
  comparison with sildenafil, 95
  definition of, 95, 177
  intraurethral. *See* MUSE
  topical (Topiglan), 147
Alprostadil alfadex (Eject), 65
American Foundation for Urologic
      Disease (AFUD), 174

American Medical Systems: inflatable penile prosthesis,
      117–118, 117*f*, 119*f*
American Urological Association,
      174
Aminobenzoate potassium (Potaba),
      77
Amitriptyline (Elavil, Endep), 18,
      27*t*
Anatomy, 2, 3*f*
Androderm, 69–70, 177
Androgel, 70–71, 177
Androgens, 68, 177
Anejaculation, 26, 55–56
  definition of, 26, 177
  treatment of, 74
Anesthesia
  complications of, 131
  definition of, 74, 177
  for electroejaculation, 74
  general, 177
  local, 177
  definition of, 50, 181
  penile arteriography with, 50
  spinal, 177
  topical, 73
Aneurysm, 135, 178
Angina, 12, 172–173, 178

Anorexia, 73, 178
Anorgasmia, 26, 56
  acquired, 56, 177
  congenital, 56, 179
  definition of, 26, 178
  treatment of, 74–75
Antidepressants, 18
  definition of, 18, 178
  for retrograde ejaculation, 73–74
  sexual dysfunction induced by, 90
Antihypertensives, 17–18, 92
Antipsychotics, 19, 90
Anxiety, 161–162
Apomorphine (Uprima), 140–141
Apomorphine SL, 65, 140–142
  comparison with sildenafil (Via-
    gra), 144–145
  how to use, 142
  side effects of, 142–144
  success rate, 142–144
Arrhythmias, 83
Arteries, 2
  definition of, 3, 178
  hardening of, 12–13, 180–181
  penile arterial bypass surgery, 23,
    136
    definition of, 23, 183
    incisions for, 137, 137f
    risks of, 138
    success rate, 137
    surgical procedure, 136–137
Arteriography, 43
  definition of, 43, 178
  penile, 49–52
Assessment
  Brief Sexual Function Inventory
    (BSFI), 36
  global assessment questionnaire
    (GAQ), 89, 180
  International Index of Erectile
    Function (IIEF), 36,
    189–191
    abbreviated questionnaire,
      193–194

physical examination, 37–38
screening, 165–166
Sexual Health Inventory for Men
  (SHIM), 36
specialized tests, 42–43
of testosterone levels, 38
Atherosclerosis, 12, 178
Autoinflation, 126, 178
Avanafil (Vivus), 146
Axial rigidity, 46–47, 178

Baclofen (Lioresal), 27t
Behavioral therapy, 72
Benign prostatic hyperplasia (BPH),
  68, 178
Benign tumors, 30–31, 178
Benzodiazepines, 19
Beta-blockers, 18
Bethanidine, 27t
Bilateral radical prostatectomy,
  88–89
Bimix (papaverine and phento-
  lamine), 64
Biopsy
  definition of, 178
  transrectal ultrasound–guided,
    71–72
Bleeding, excessive, 131
Blood pressure
  high, 17–18, 83
  low, 81, 181
    orthostatic hypotension, 141,
      183
    and PDE-5 inhibitors, 81
Books, 175
BPH. See Benign prostatic hyperpla-
  sia
Brief Sexual Function Inventory
  (BSFI), 36
Brompheniramine maleate
  (Bromfed), 28t
BSFI. See Brief Sexual Function
  Inventory
Buccal testosterone therapy, 71

Butterfly needles, 49, 178
Bypass surgery, penile arterial, 23, 136
  definition of, 23, 183
  incisions for, 137, 137f
  risks of, 138
  success rate, 137
  surgical procedure, 136–137

Carbamazepine (Tegretol), 20
Catheter, 50
  definition of, 50, 178
  Foley catheter, 121–122, 180
Causes of erectile dysfunction, 9–20
Caverject. *See also* Alprostadil
  cavernosometry with, 48–49
  definition of, 65, 178
  injection therapy with, 64, 100, 177
    comparison with sildenafil, 95
    dosage and volume calculations for, 106t
    points to keep in mind, 105
    risks of, 108
Cavermap Surgical Aid (Uromed), 149
Cavernosography, 43, 49, 178
Cavernosometry, 48–49, 178
Central nervous system, 141, 178
cGMP, 14, 178
Chest pain, 173–174
Chlordiazepoxide (Librium), 27t
Chlorimipramine, 27t
Chlorpheniramine (Chlor-Trimeton), 28t
Chlorpromazine (Thorazine), 27t, 55
Chlorthalidone (Hygroton), 18
Cholesterol, 13, 178
Cialis. *See* Tadalafil
Cimetidine (Tagamet), 19, 84
Clarithromycin (Biaxin), 84
Clofibrate (Atomid-S), 19
Clomipramine (Anafranil), 18, 27t, 72–73
Clonazepam (Klonopin), 19

Clonidine (Catapres), 18
Colchicine, 77
Combined therapies, 151–153
Communication
  with insurance clerks, 171
  talking about erectile dysfunction, 155–175
  talking with your wife/partner, 159–160
  visits with partners, 166–167
  with your doctor, 164–166
Complications, 116, 179
Congenital anorgasmia, 56, 179
Congestive heart failure, 68, 81, 179
Corona, 46, 179
Corpora cavernosa, 2, 179
Corpus spongiosum, 2, 179
"Couples problems," 166–167

Delayed ejaculation, 26, 179
Depression, 9, 161–162, 179
Desipramine (Norpramine), 73–74
Detumescence, 24, 179
Diabetes mellitus, 13–14
  definition of, 13, 179
  insulin-dependent, 14, 181
  non–insulin-dependent, 14, 182
  penile injection therapy with, 107
  success rates for sildenafil in men with, 87
Diagnosis, 34, 179
Dialysis, 87
Diazepam (Valium), 19
Digital rectal examination (DRE), 66, 179
Digoxin, 19–20
Disease, 7, 179
Doctors
  Bob's comment on, 164–165
  communicating with, 164–166
  visits with wife/partner, 166–167
  who to see, 160–161
Doppler ultrasonography, 43
  definition of, 43, 179
  penile, 47–48

Index

Double-blind studies, 146, 179
Doxazosin (Cardura), 18, 177
  combined therapy with, 152–153
  dosing recommendations for
     PDE-5 inhibitors in men
     taking, 83–84
DRE. *See* Digital rectal examination
Drugs. *See* Medications; *specific drugs
    by name*

EBRT. *See* External-beam radiation
  therapy
Economic impacts, 8
Edex (alprostadil alfadex). *See also*
  Alprostadil
  cavernosometry with, 48–49
  definition of, 65, 179
  injection therapy with, 64, 100,
    177
    comparison with sildenafil, 95
    dosage and volume calculations
     for, 106*t*
    points to keep in mind, 105
    risks of, 108
Efficacy, 98, 179
Ejaculate, 189
Ejaculation, 21, 25–26. *See also* Anejaculation
  definition of, 21, 179
  delayed, 26, 179
  electroejaculation, 74, 179
  medications associated with
    impairment of, 27*t*
  medications that affect, 27*t*–28*t*
  premature, 25–26, 54
    definition of, 25, 183–184
    treatment of, 72–73
  retrograde, 26, 54–55
    definition of, 26, 184
    treatment of, 73–74
Ejaculatory duct, 55, 179
Ejaculatory dysfunction, 25, 179
Electroejaculation, 74, 179
Ellsworth, Pamela, vi–vii
Embolization, 75, 180

Emission, 24, 180
EMLA gels, 73
Encore, 110
Enzymes, 67, 180
Ephedrine, 28*t*, 73–74
Epsilon aminocaproic acid (Amicar),
  27*t*
Erectile dysfunction, 5–7
  and aging, 20–21
  assessment of
    multidimensional scale for,
     189–191
    questionnaire for, 193–194
  causes of, 9–20
  as "couples problem," 166–167
  curability of, 22–24
  current options for, 62–65
  definition of, 5, 180
  diagnosis of, 34
  economic impact of, 8
  evaluation of, 33–51, 35*f*
  goal-oriented approach to, 35*f*, 39
  iatrogenic causes of, 63
  incidence of, 8
  living with, 155–175
  medications associated with,
    10*t*–11*t*
  medications that cause, 17–20
  neurologic conditions that cause, 9
  NIH definition of, 5–6
  oral therapy for, 62, 79–80
  other conditions that cause, 13–17
  in Peyronie's disease, 60
  prevalence of, 7–8, 7*f*
  prevention of, 22
  psychogenic, 17
  psychogenic causes of, 17, 64
  risk factors, 63
  screening for, 165–166
  talking about, 155–175
  therapies under investigation,
    145–151
  treatment of, 22–24, 35*f*, 61–153
  vascular conditions that cause,
    12–13

women's response to, 164
Erection
definition of, 2, 180
mechanism of, 2–4, 4f
neurologic mechanism of, 14, 15f
nocturnal, 6, 170–171, 182
normal, 2–5
prolonged, 56, 184
testosterone and, 39
Erosion
definition of, 132, 180
with penile prosthesis, 132–133
Erythromycin (E-mycin), 84
Examination, physical, 37–38
Experimental treatments, 22
definition of, 22, 180
investigational treatments, 145–151
External-beam radiation therapy (EBRT), 12, 88, 180

Famotidine (Pepcid), 19
FDA. See Food and Drug Administration
Fibrosis, penile, 109
Financial assistance, 169–170
Fluoxetine (Prozac), 18, 27t
and anorgasmia, 74–75
for premature ejaculation, 73
Fluphenazine (Prolixin), 19
Fluvoxamine (Luvox), 18
Foley catheter, 121–122, 180
Food and Drug Administration (FDA), 29, 180
Forskolin, 148–149

GAQ. See Global assessment questionnaire
Gel
topical anesthetic, 73
topical testosterone, 70–71
Gemfibrozil (Lopid), 19
Gender, 165, 180
Gender issues, 165
Gene therapy, 151, 180

Genitalia, 37, 180
Genitourinary tract, 24, 180
Glans, 2, 180
Glans droop, 133
Global assessment questionnaire (GAQ), 89, 180
Glycosylated end-products, 14, 180
Glycosylated hemoglobin, 87, 180
Goserelin (Zoladex), 20
Groin, 50, 180
Guanethidine sulfate (Ismelin), 27t
Gynecomastia, 37, 180

Haloperidol (Haldol), 27t
Hardening of the arteries, 12–13, 180–181
HDL. See High-density lipoprotein
Health insurance, 171–172
Heart failure, congestive, 68, 81, 179
Hematoma
definition of, 108, 181
with penile injection therapy, 108
with vacuum device, 116
Hemodialysis, 15–16
Hemoglobin, glycosylated, 87, 180
Hexamethonium, 27t
High blood pressure, 83
High-density lipoprotein (HDL), 13, 181
High-flow priapism, 56–57, 75, 181
History, 34, 181
Hormones, 30, 185
Hypercholesterolemia, 8, 181
Hyperprolactinemia, 17, 181
Hypertension, 17–18, 181
Hypogonadism, 17, 181
Hypotension
definition of, 81, 181
orthostatic, 141, 183
and PDE-5 inhibitors, 81

Iatrogenic causes, 63, 181
IIEF. See International Index of Erectile Function
Imipramine (Tofranil), 18, 27t–28t

Implants. *See* Penile prosthesis
Impotence. *See* Erectile dysfunction
Incidence, 8, 181
Indications, 66, 181
Indinavir (Crixivan), 84
Infection, 132
Inflatable penile prosthesis, 117–118, 117*f*
 three-piece, 118, 119*f*
 two-piece, 118, 118*f*
Infrapubic incision, 122
Injection therapy
 Bob's comment on, 100–101
 current options, 64
 dosage and volume calculations for, 106*t*
 intracavernous, 99, 181
  combined with doxazosin, 152–153
  comparison with sildenafil, 95
  FDA-approved chemicals for, 100
  investigational treatments, 148–149
 penile, 99–100
  candidates for, 101–102
  dose required for, 107
  how to use, 102–106
  risks of, 107–110
  success rates, 106
 points to keep in mind, 104–106
 proper location of injection, 103, 104*f*
 with prostaglandin E$_1$, 106*t*
Inpatient stays, 121, 181
Insulin-dependent diabetes mellitus, 14, 181
Insurance, 171–172
Intercourse. *See* Sexual intercourse
International Index of Erectile Function (IIEF), 36, 189–191
 abbreviated questionnaire, 193–194
International Society of Impotence Research, 174

Interposition, 149, 181
Interposition sural nerve grafting, 149–151
Intracavernous injection therapy, 99. *See also* Penile injection therapy
 combined with doxazosin, 152–153
 comparison with sildenafil, 95
 definition of, 181
 FDA-approved chemicals for, 100
Intracavernous pressure, 49, 181
Intramuscular (IM) testosterone therapy
 definition of, 67, 181
 parenteral, 68–69
 recommended dose, 69
Intraurethral alprostadil. *See* MUSE
Investigational treatments, 145–151
 experimental treatments, 22, 180
 gene therapies, 151
 injection therapies, 148–149
 oral therapies, 146–147
 surgical therapies, 149–151
 topical therapies, 147–148
Ischemia
 definition of, 116, 181
 penile, 116, 133–134
Ischemic optic neuropathy, nonarteritic (NAION), 93–94, 182
Itraconazole (Sporanox), 84

Ketoconazole (Nizoral), 84

L-Arginine, 146–147
Laboratory tests, 41–42
Leukemia, 57, 181
Leuprolide (Lupron), 20
Levitra. *See* Vardenafil
LH. *See* Luteinizing hormone
Libido, 20, 25
 decreased, 30–31
 definition of, 20, 181
Lifestyle changes, 63
Lindisomine, 148

Lipoprotein, high-density (HDL), 13, 181
Liver function enzymes, 67
Liver toxicity, 109–110
Local anesthesia, 50, 177, 181
Lorazepam (Ativan), 19
Lovastatin (Mevacor), 19
Low blood pressure, 81, 181
  orthostatic hypotension, 141, 183
  and PDE-5 inhibitors, 81
Low-flow priapism, 57, 75, 181
Luteinizing hormone (LH), 30, 181–182
Lymph node dissection, retroperitoneal, 55, 185

Marijuana, 20
Mechanical therapy, 64
Medicare, 171
Medications. *See also specific medications by name*
  associated with erectile dysfunction, 10t–11t
  associated with impairment of ejaculation, 27t
  over-the-counter treatments, 168–169
  to promote seminal emission, 28t
  that affect ejaculation, 27t–28t
  that cause erectile dysfunction, 17–20
Mentor Urology, 110
Mesoridazine (Serentil), 55
Methadone (Dolophine), 27t
Monoamine oxidase inhibitors, 102
Morbidity, 62, 182
Mortality, 62, 182
MUSE (intraurethral alprostadil), 95–96, 177
  candidates for, 96–97
  combined with sildenafil (Viagra), 152
  definition of, 95, 182
  doses, 98
  efficacy of, 98
  how to use, 97–98, 97f
  insertion of, 97–98, 97f
  side effects of, 99
  success rate, 98–99
Myths, 158, 182

NAION. *See* Nonarteritic ischemic optic neuropathy
Naproxen (Naprosyn), 27t
National Institutes of Health (NIH), 5–6
Necrosis, penile, 133–134
Needles, butterfly, 49, 178
Nelfinavir (Viracept), 84
Nerve grafting, interposition, 149–151
Nerves, 4–5, 182
Neurologic conditions, 9
Neurotransmitters, 5, 182
Nitrates, 81, 82t, 182
Nitric oxide, 14, 182
Nitroglycerin, 81, 172–173, 182
Nocturnal erections, 6, 170–171, 182
Nocturnal penile tumescence (NPT) studies, 42, 44–46, 182
Nonarteritic ischemic optic neuropathy (NAION), 93–94, 182
Non–insulin-dependent diabetes mellitus, 14, 182
Noninvasive procedures, 182
NPT studies. *See* Nocturnal penile tumescence studies

Objectivity, 6, 182
Occlusion, 48, 75, 182
Occult prostate cancer, 66
Opiates, 20
Optic neuropathy, nonarteritic ischemic (NAION), 93–94, 182
Oral therapy, 62
  current options, 64
  definition of, 62, 182
  investigational, 146–147
  with PDE-5 inhibitors, 80–84

for premature ejaculation, 72–73
testosterone therapy, 68
Orchiectomy, 20, 183
Organ, 24, 183
Organizations, 174
Orgasm, 26, 183
Orgasmic dysfunction, 26, 183
Orthostatic hypotension, 141, 183
Osbon, 110
Over-the-counter treatments,
168–169

Pain
with penile injection therapy, 108
with penile prosthesis, 134
perineal, 134
with vacuum device, 115
Palpation, 37, 183
Papaverine, 64
bimix (papaverine and phentolamine), 64
triple P (phentolamine,
prostaglandin, and papaverine), 64, 100
in combination with sildenafil,
152
comparison with sildenafil, 95
risks with, 109
Parenteral (intramuscular) testosterone therapy, 68–69, 183
Pargyline (Eutonyl), 27t
Paroxetine (Paxil), 18–19, 27t, 73
Partner/wife
female response to male erectile
dysfunction, 164
talking with, 159–161
visits with, 166–167
Patch therapy, 69–70
PDE-5 inhibitors. See Phosphodiesterase type 5 inhibitors
Pelvis, 5, 183
Penile arterial bypass surgery, 23, 136
definition of, 23, 183
incisions for, 137, 137f
risks of, 138

success rate, 137
surgical procedure, 136–137
Penile arteriography, 49–52
Penile Doppler ultrasonography,
47–48
Penile fibrosis, 109
Penile injection therapy, 99–100
candidates for, 101–102
dose required for, 107
how to use, 102–106
risks of, 107–110
success rates, 106
Penile ischemia
with penile prosthesis, 133–134
with vacuum device, 116
Penile length, decreased, 131
Penile necrosis, 133–134
Penile prosthesis, 64, 116–119
advantages of, 129
autoinflation of, 126, 135
Bob's comments on, 124–125,
127–129, 135–136, 171
candidates for, 119–121
complications of, 130–136
intraoperative, 130–131
postoperative, 131–135
definition of, 64, 183
disadvantages of, 135–136
for erectile dysfunction with Peyronie's disease, 79
health insurance coverage for,
171–172
how to use, 121–122
indications for, 120–121
inflatable, 117–118, 117f
three-piece, 118, 119f
two-piece, 118, 118f
mechanical problems, 134–135
mechanics of, 121–122, 125
migration of, 132–133, 182
placement of, 121–122
hospital and postoperative
course, 125–128
surgical approaches to, 122
risks of, 130–136

semi-rigid, 117, 117*f*
success rate for, 129
success rate for sildenafil in men
    with, 88
Penis, 2
    anatomy of, 2, 3*f*
    curvature of, of Peyronie's disease
        residual, after prosthesis place-
            ment, 131, 134
        surgical treatment of, 78–79
    definition of, 2, 183
Penoscrotal incision, 122
Perineal pain, 134
Perineum, 22, 183
Perphenazine (Etrafon), 27*t*
Peyronie's disease, 12–13, 57–59
    definition of, 13, 183
    erectile dysfunction in, 60
    evaluation of, 59–60
    penile curvature of
        residual after prosthesis place-
            ment, 131, 134
        surgical treatment of, 78–79
    treatment of, 76–79
Phenelzine sulfate (Nardil), 27*t*
Phenobarbitol, 20
Phenoxybenzamiine hydrochloride
        (Dibenzyline), 27*t*, 55
Phentolamine, 27*t*, 55
    bimix (papaverine and phento-
        lamine), 64
    triple P (phentolamine,
        prostaglandin, and papaver-
        ine), 64, 100
    in combination with sildenafil,
        152
    comparison with sildenafil, 95
    risks with, 109
Phenylpropanolamine (Entex,
        Hycomine, Profen), 28*t*
Phenytoin (Dilantin), 20
Phosphodiesterase type 5 (PDE-5),
        80, 183
Phosphodiesterase type 5 (PDE-5)
        inhibitors

candidates for oral therapy, 80–84
    cautions, 81–83
    comparison with other therapies
        for erectile dysfunction,
        94–95
    contraindications to, 81
    definition of, 79, 183
    dosing recommendations, 83–84
    for erectile dysfunction, 79–80
    how to use, 84–85
    investigational therapies, 146
    medications that increase levels of,
        84
    side effects of, 90–94
    success rate, 85–86
    use of, 84–85
Physical examination, 37–38
Physicians
    Bob's comment on, 164–165
    communicating with, 164–166
    who to see, 160–161
Physiologic functioning, 183
Physiologic testosterone levels, 69
Pituitary adenoma, 9, 30–31, 183
Pituitary gland, 30, 183
Placebo, 76, 183
Plaque formation, 109
Polycythemia, 67, 183
Post-T-Vac, 110
Postage stamp test, 44
Pravastatin (Pravachol), 19
Prazosin hydrochloride (Minipress),
        27*t*, 55, 153
Premature ejaculation, 54
    definition of, 25, 183–184
    diagnostic criteria for, 54, 184
    treatment of, 72–73
Prevalence, 7–8, 7*f*, 8, 184
Priapism, 56–57
    definition of, 56, 184
    high-flow, 56–57, 75, 181
    with intracavernous injection ther-
        apy, 103
    low-flow, 57, 75, 181

with penile injection therapy,
108–109
treatment of, 75–76
types of, 75
Primary care providers, 160–161
Primidone (Mysoline), 20
Prolactin, 19, 184
Propranolol (Indeval), 18
Prostaglandin. *See* Triple P (phentolamine, prostaglandin, and
papaverine)
Prostaglandin E₁
definition of, 65, 184
dosage and volume calculations
for, 106*t*
injection therapy with, 64
Prostate, 55, 184
Prostate cancer, occult, 66
Prostatectomy
radical
bilateral, 88–89
definition of, 89, 184
interposition sural nerve grafting
during, 149–151
transurethral (TURP), 54–55, 186
Prosthesis, 24
definition of, 24, 184
penile. *See* Penile prosthesis
Protease inhibitors, 84
Protriptyline (Concordin), 18
Pseudoephedrine hydrochloride
(Sudafed), 28*t*, 73–74
Psychogenic causes, 17, 64, 184
Psychogenic erectile dysfunction, 17
Psychosocial factors, 63, 158–159
Publications, 175

Quality of life, 62, 184

Radial rigidity, 46, 184
Radiation therapy, 12
definition of, 12, 184
external-beam (EBRT), 12, 88,
180
Radical prostatectomy

bilateral, 88–89
definition of, 89, 184
interposition sural nerve grafting
during, 149–151
Randomized studies, 77, 184
Ranitidine (Zantac), 19
Rapid eye movement (REM), 45,
184
Rapid eye movement (REM) sleep,
45
Rectal examination, digital (DRE),
66, 179
Red blood cells, 39, 184
REM. *See* Rapid eye movement
"Rescue" procedures, 185
Reserpine (Serpasil), 27*t*
Resistance
definition of, 184
venous, 43, 48
Resources, 174–175
Retinitis pigmentosa, 83
Retrograde ejaculation, 26, 54–55,
184
Retroperitoneal lymph node dissec-
tion, 55, 185
Rigidity
axial, 46–47, 178
radial, 46, 184
RigiScan (Timm Medical Technolo-
gies), 46–47
Risk, 63, 185
Risk factors, 63
Ritonavir (Norvir), 84

Salvage procedures, 132, 185
Saquinavir (Fortovase), 84
Scarring, 131
Schwarz Pharma, 179
Screening, 165–166
Scrotum, 22, 185
Selective serotonin reuptake
inhibitors (SSRIs), 18–19,
27*t*
definition of, 18, 185
for premature ejaculation, 73

Self-doubt, 161–162
Semen
    definition of, 21, 185
    drugs used to promote emission of, 28t
Sertraline (Zoloft), 18, 27t, 73
Sex hormones, 30, 185
Sex therapy, 167–168
Sexual activity, 189
Sexual desire, 191
Sexual dysfunction, 6
    and aging, 20–21
    Brief Sexual Function Inventory (BSFI), 36
    definition of, 6, 24–26, 185
    types of, 53–60
    in women, 26–29, 28f
Sexual Health Inventory for Men (SHIM), 36
Sexual intercourse
    chest pain during, 173–174
    definition of, 189
Sexual response cycle, 63, 185
Sexual stimulation, 189
SHIM. See Sexual Health Inventory for Men
Sickle cell disease/sickle cell trait, 57, 185
Side effects, 19, 185
Signs, 37, 185
Sildenafil (Viagra), 64, 79
    combined with intracavernous injection therapy, 152
    combined with intraurethral alprostadil (MUSE), 152
    combined with triple P injection therapy, 152
    comparison with apomorphine, 144–145
    comparison with other therapies for erectile dysfunction, 94–95
    contraindications to, 172–173
    definition of, 64, 185
    dosing recommendations, 83

effects on female sexual dysfunction, 29
for men who have undergone EBRT, 88
for men with inflatable penile prostheses, 88
and nitroglycerin, 172–173
for patients on dialysis, 87
for patients with diabetes mellitus, 87
for patients with spinal cord injury or spina bifida, 87
projected sales of, 8
after radical prostatectomy, 88–89
rare side effects of, 93–94
side effects of, 91, 92t
success rates, 85, 86t, 87–90
use of, 84–85
Sinusoids, 4, 185
Sleep
    nocturnal erections, 6, 170–171, 182
    nocturnal penile tumescence (NPT) studies, 42, 44–46, 182
    rapid eye movement (REM) sleep, 45
SLx-2101 (SurfaceLogix), 146
Smoking, 16
Snap-Gauge test, 44
Somnolence, 143–144, 185
Specialized tests, 42–43
Spina bifida, 87
Spinal anesthesia, 177
Spinal cord injury, 87, 107
SSRIs. See Selective serotonin reuptake inhibitors
Stanley, Bob, vii–viii
Stress, 161–162
Striant, 71, 185
Subcoronal incision, 122
Subjectivity, 6, 185
"Sugar pills," 183
Supplemental testosterone, 65–66

Supraphysiologic functioning, 68, 185

Supraphysiologic testosterone levels, 68–69

Sural nerve grafting, interposition, 149–151

Surgery, 65
investigational therapies, 149–151
penile bypass surgery, 136–137
penile prosthesis placement, 122, 130–131
for Peyronie's disease, 78–79
venous ligation surgery, 138–140, 187

Symptoms, 7, 185

Syncope, 96, 185

Synergist, 110

Tachyphylaxis, 94, 186

Tadalafil (Cialis), 64, 79
definition of, 65, 186
dosing recommendations, 84
for patients with spinal cord injury, 87
rare side effects of, 93–94
side effects of, 91, 92*t*
success rates, 86, 88
use of, 84–85

Talking about erectile dysfunction, 155–175
Bob's comments on, 156, 159, 161
key issues, 157–158
with your wife/partner, 159–161

Tamoxifen, 77

Tamsulosin (Flowmax), 177
dosing recommendations for PDE-5 inhibitors in men taking, 83–84
retrograde ejaculation and, 55

Terazosin (Hytrin), 83–84, 177

Tesosterone patch therapy, 69–70

Testes, 30, 186

Testim, 70–71, 186

Testoderm, 69–70, 186

Testoderm TTS, 69–70

Testosterone, 25
assessing, 38
definition of, 25, 186
effects on erections, 39
physiologic levels, 69
supraphysiologic levels, 68–69

Testosterone supplementation, 65–66

Testosterone therapy
benefits and risks of, 66–68
buccal, 71
intramuscular (IM)
definition of, 67, 181
recommended dose, 69
monitoring, 71–72
oral, 68
parenteral (intramuscular), 68–69
transdermal, 67, 69–71
types of, 68–71

The Impotence Association, 174

Thiazides (hydrochlorothiazide), 27*t*

Thioridazine (Mellaril), 19, 27*t*, 55

Thiothixene (Navane), 19

Timm Medical Technologies, 46–47, 110

Tissue
benign prostate, 67
definition of, 67, 186

Topical therapies
anesthetic gels for premature ejaculation, 73
investigational treatments, 147–148
testosterone therapy, 70–71

Transdermal therapy
definition of, 186
testosterone therapy, 67, 69–71

Transrectal therapy, 186

Transrectal ultrasound, 186

Transrectal ultrasound–guided biopsy, 71–72

Transurethral prostatectomy (TURP), 54–55, 186

Trazodone, 65
definition of, 66, 186

Index

investigational treatment, 147
Treatment, 61–153
  current options, 62–65
  psychosocial factors, 158–159
Trifluoroperazine (Stelazine), 27t
Triflupromazine (Vespein), 55
Triple P (phentolamine,
    prostaglandin, and papaver-
    ine), 64, 100
  in combination with sildenafil, 152
  comparison with sildenafil, 95
  risks with, 109
Tumescence, 42, 186
  nocturnal penile tumescence
    (NPT) studies, 42, 44–46,
    182
Tunica albuginea, 2, 186
TURP. See Transurethral prostatec-
    tomy

Ultrasound, 43
  definition of, 43, 186
  Doppler ultrasonography, 43
    definition of, 43, 179
    penile, 47–48
  transrectal, 71–72, 186
Urethra, 2–3, 186
Urologists, 24, 160–161, 165
  American Urological Association,
    174
  definition of, 24, 186
US TOO International, Inc., 174

Vacuum devices, 64, 110–112, 111f
  Bob's comments on, 111–112, 115
  candidates for, 112–113
  comparison with sildenafil, 95
  complications of, 116
  definition of, 64, 186–187
  how to use, 111f, 113
  over-the-counter devices, 169
  principles of, 110
  side effects of, 115–116

success and satisfaction rates,
    113–115
Vardenafil (Levitra), 64, 79
  definition of, 65, 187
  dosing recommendations, 83
  for patients with spinal cord injury,
    87
  side effects of, 91, 92t, 93–94
  success rate, 85
  use of, 84–85
Vas deferens, 56, 187
Vascular conditions, 12–13
Vasoactive intestinal peptide, 148
Vasospasm, 12, 187
Vasovagal attacks, 144, 187
Veins, 2–3, 187
Venous leak, 23, 187
Venous ligation surgery, 23–24,
    138–139
  candidates for, 139
  definition of, 23, 187
  risks of, 139–140
  success rate, 139–140
  surgical procedure, 140
Venous resistance, 43, 48
Verapamil, 77–78
Viagra. See Sildenafil
Vitamin E, 76

Warfarin (Coumadin), 102
Wasting, 57–58
Web sites, 175
Wife/partner
  doctor visits with, 166–167
  talking with, 159–161
Women
  response to male erectile dysfunc-
    tion, 164
  sexual dysfunction in, 26–29, 28f

X-rays, 49, 187

Yohimbine, 65–66, 145, 187